Acclaim for *The Long COVID Sur*

"This is the Long COVID book that the world needs—a practical, authoritative, compassionate, and ultimately hopeful guide to a difficult condition, written by the people who understand it best. So many long-haulers have faced their illness alone and unheard; none ever need to do so again."**—Ed Yong, *New York Times*-bestselling author of *An Immense World* and Pulitzer Prize-winning journalist**

"*The Long COVID Survival Guide* is not only a moving and helpful compilation of stories but a necessary one, given how many lives Long COVID will touch as coronavirus infections accumulate. It brings practical and emotional support to those who are struggling to navigate a scary new reality. *The Long COVID Survival Guide* is not just for patients but their loved ones, friends, colleagues— in short, all of us. I wish I'd had this book when I first got sick with a similar condition a decade ago!"**—Meghan O'Rourke, *New York Times*-bestselling author of *The Invisible Kingdom***

"This book is a much-needed antidote to the isolation of Long COVID. Drawing on their personal experiences, the authors offer important advice on getting properly diagnosed, dealing with medical racism, finding community support, and more—all while reminding you that you are not alone on the journey to recovery."**—Oni Blackstock, MD, MHS, founder and executive director of Health Justice**

"A gem of a book that provides accessible, vital, and insightful information delivered in a way that is welcoming, kind, and encouraging—and from people who know best about this perplexing condition. Beautifully done, you can feel the caring in each page . . . and readily appreciate the wisdom. An amazing accomplishment to have produced such a gift to all those who are suffering— and all those who care about them."**—Harlan Krumholz, MD, SM, professor of medicine, Yale University, and director of the Yale Center for Outcomes Research and Evaluation**

"There is still a lot to research and learn in order to understand the mechanisms behind Long COVID and the mostly unseen public health crisis it has caused. This book tells its origin story through the personal experiences of a community of patients, empowered to be their own advocates. It shows that there's strength, support, answers, and hope in collective knowledge and shared experiences with managing a complex condition. It informs about the evolving research on Long COVID and emphasizes the importance of collaboration between patients and health care providers. Above all, it affirms the power of a robust community to bring us closer to improving care and overall health and well-being in the pandemic's aftermath."—**Michelle Williams, SM, ScD, dean of the faculty and professor of epidemiology, Harvard T. H. Chan School of Public Health**

"*The Long COVID Survival Guide* centers the true experts on Long COVID: patients who, from the earliest days of the pandemic, have offered each other validation, practical advice, and solidarity in navigating a biased medical system. Their hard-won wisdom is essential reading for anyone who cares about building a better society for chronically ill people."—**Maya Dusenbery, author of *Doing Harm: The Truth About How Bad Medicine and Lazy Science Leave Women Dismissed, Misdiagnosed, and Sick***

"*The Long COVID Survival Guide* is an urgent, informative, deeply personal collection of essays and interviews from people living with Long COVID, their caregivers, and advocates. It's a thorough, lucid, user-friendly handbook, designed to help COVID long-haulers understand their symptoms and navigate the often-baffling health care system so they can get the care they deserve. It gives hard-earned peer-group advice, lists steps to take and resources to make use of, and links to the international networks of information and support that long-haulers, the ultimate experts on Long COVID, have had to construct themselves. But its chapters also chronicle an ongoing worldwide epidemic, the spotty medical and governmental response to it, and the cost to individuals and their loved ones—stories that will engage anyone who has had to endure the twists and turns of this epidemic without end."—**Jim Eigo, ACT UP NY**

THE
LONG
COVID
SURVIVAL
GUIDE

How to Take Care of Yourself and What Comes Next

Edited by Fiona Lowenstein

THE EXPERIMENT

NEW YORK

The Experiment, LLC
220 East 23rd Street, Suite 600
New York, NY 10010-4658
theexperimentpublishing.com

The Experiment's books are available at special discounts when purchased in bulk for premiums and sales promotions as well as for fundraising or educational use. For details, contact us at info@theexperimentpublishing.com.

Library of Congress Cataloging-in-Publication Data

Names: Lowenstein, Fiona, editor.
Title: The long COVID survival guide : how to take care of yourself and what comes next / edited by Fiona Lowenstein.
Description: New York : The Experiment, 2022. | Includes bibliographical references and index. | Summary: "The first patient-to-patient guide for people living with Long COVID, with answers and reassurance to guide readers through issues like getting diagnosed, dealing with symptoms, and caring for their mental health"-- Provided by publisher.
Identifiers: LCCN 2022027166 (print) | LCCN 2022027167 (ebook) | ISBN 9781615199105 (paperback) | ISBN 9781615199112 (ebook)
Subjects: LCSH: COVID-19 (Disease)--Complications--Popular works. | COVID-19 (Disease)--Patients--Medical care--Popular works. | COVID-19 (Disease)--Psychological aspects--Popular works. | COVID-19 (Disease)--Diagnosis--Popular works. | Chronically ill--Care--Popular works.
Classification: LCC RA644.C67 L69 2022 (print) | LCC RA644.C67 (ebook) | DDC 616.2/414--dc23/eng/20220722
LC record available at https://lccn.loc.gov/2022027166
LC ebook record available at https://lccn.loc.gov/2022027167

ISBN 978-1-61519-910-5
Ebook ISBN 978-1-61519-911-2

Cover and text design by Beth Bugler

Manufactured in the United States of America

First printing November 2022
10 9 8 7 6 5 4 3

*To the millions missing**

*The #MillionsMissing campaign was created by ME/CFS advocacy organization #MEAction to recognize the millions of people who have been sidelined from society due to inadequate support for people with complex chronic illnesses—and the millions of dollars missing from research into ME/CFS and other post-viral and infection-initiated diseases. To learn more, visit millionsmissing. meaction.net.

Contents

All You Need Is One Person

The Birth of a Patient Community (and What to Expect from This Book)

Fiona Lowenstein

Part I: Just in Case . . .

It was March 10, 2020, and a warm breeze was starting to soften the cold New York City air—"fake spring," we called it, because true New Yorkers know spring can't really be counted on until at least May. Still, I remember feeling excited about the dawning change of seasons as I hurried home from my afternoon fitness class to meet a friend for dinner.

At the yoga and fitness studio where I taught part-time, people were just starting to talk about the new virus spreading in China, and now Italy, but no one seemed especially concerned. By March 10, at least one case of community spread had been confirmed in New York City, and as an added precaution, I'd started carrying hand sanitizer and antibacterial wipes. I wouldn't be doing any hands-on adjustments, I explained to my students—just in case.

Just in case was a phrase that had started increasingly tickling at the back of my brain that month—a fleeting feeling of fear that briefly caused me to wonder if I should stock up on toilet paper or cancel my dinner plans, but which I quickly combated with the anti-anxiety mantras I embraced to manage my fast-paced city life. So, I didn't cancel my plans. Instead, I repeated something I'd heard that morning on my meditation app: I told myself to stop "what if"-ing. Then, I hurried home, showered, and prepared to host my friend, Sabrina, for dinner.

Sabrina and I had met in a college feminist comedy troupe, but in many ways, it felt like we'd known each other our whole lives. We were both only children, raised in New York City, who'd lived in Hell's Kitchen as kids and attended a mix of public and private schools on financial aid. At college, we shared a major, extracurricular interests, and even the same scholarship benefactor. After graduating, I'd launched Body Politic, a queer feminist wellness collective and events series, and Sabrina had quickly come on board as a co-leader, organizing events and helping to launch a Body Politic blog. On that particular Tuesday night, we planned to do what we loved: cook, eat, and brainstorm new creative ideas.

All You Need Is One Person

The Birth of a Patient Community (and What to Expect from This Book)

Fiona Lowenstein

Part I: Just in Case . . .

It was March 10, 2020, and a warm breeze was starting to soften the cold New York City air—"fake spring," we called it, because true New Yorkers know spring can't really be counted on until at least May. Still, I remember feeling excited about the dawning change of seasons as I hurried home from my afternoon fitness class to meet a friend for dinner.

At the yoga and fitness studio where I taught part-time, people were just starting to talk about the new virus spreading in China, and now Italy, but no one seemed especially concerned. By March 10, at least one case of community spread had been confirmed in New York City, and as an added precaution, I'd started carrying hand sanitizer and antibacterial wipes. I wouldn't be doing any hands-on adjustments, I explained to my students—just in case.

Just in case was a phrase that had started increasingly tickling at the back of my brain that month—a fleeting feeling of fear that briefly caused me to wonder if I should stock up on toilet paper or cancel my dinner plans, but which I quickly combated with the anti-anxiety mantras I embraced to manage my fast-paced city life. So, I didn't cancel my plans. Instead, I repeated something I'd heard that morning on my meditation app: I told myself to stop "what if"-ing. Then, I hurried home, showered, and prepared to host my friend, Sabrina, for dinner.

Sabrina and I had met in a college feminist comedy troupe, but in many ways, it felt like we'd known each other our whole lives. We were both only children, raised in New York City, who'd lived in Hell's Kitchen as kids and attended a mix of public and private schools on financial aid. At college, we shared a major, extracurricular interests, and even the same scholarship benefactor. After graduating, I'd launched Body Politic, a queer feminist wellness collective and events series, and Sabrina had quickly come on board as a co-leader, organizing events and helping to launch a Body Politic blog. On that particular Tuesday night, we planned to do what we loved: cook, eat, and brainstorm new creative ideas.

When Sabrina arrived, we talked about the coronavirus, discussing possible outcomes, and considering ways we—as young, seemingly "healthy" people—could support others at greater risk. We agreed that this health crisis would be important to address through Body Politic's work. But after several hours of FaceTime meetings with other members of our team and more than one course of our homemade cucumber salad and meatballs, Sabrina suddenly became very pale. She said she felt sick. *Just in case*, we cut our evening short, and Sabrina went home to rest.

Those of us who became sick with COVID-19 in March and April of 2020 in the United States often call ourselves "first-wavers," even though we now know there were waves of American patients that predated the confirmed cases that spring. We use this term because it helps us identify one another and speak about the unique experiences we had as some of the first people to know we'd been infected.

Getting sick with COVID-19 in March 2020 in New York City was not an unusual experience (so many people had been infected by the time I was hospitalized that health care staff told me the virus was likely circulating on the subway and in the streets). But it was an isolating experience. News headlines and public health agencies told us that as young people without known comorbidities, we had nothing to fear. I trusted this advice, until I couldn't.

On the evening of March 13, 2020, I began to develop a fever and headache. The following day, I had a cough. Two days later, I was struggling to breathe. A borough away in Brooklyn, Sabrina's case was also progressing. But, unlike me, Sabrina didn't have a trusted primary care provider. We both had to fight to access telehealth appointments—appointments that proved useless in providing us with information or treatment—but I had a PCP who'd known me for years. When I began to rapidly decline, she urged me to seek help at an emergency room and called ahead to let them know I was coming.

I was hospitalized because I had severe shortness of breath. But there are other factors that likely helped me get admitted: I had a doctor vouching for me, I was accompanied by my partner who advocated for me, and I went to the hospital a couple of days before it became completely overwhelmed. I am also white, thin, and young, and I did not have a history of preexisting conditions, chronic illness, or disabilities. Having grown up with spotty health insurance and a parent with a preexisting health condition, I was somewhat aware of these privileges and the ways the medical system can work. I remember making a conscious choice to wear my Yale sweatshirt to the emergency room in the hope it would signal some kind of power or wealth. In reality, I was a freelance journalist, dog-walker, and fitness instructor without employer-based health insurance or a wealthy or powerful family to intervene on my behalf. Still, I was better off than so many.

My time in the hospital was short, and I won't dwell on it here, both because my story has been told many times and because hospitalization in the acute phase is not an experience all Long COVID patients share. Many others in this situation, like Sabrina, were unable to be hospitalized because—despite debilitating symptoms—they did not exhibit shortness of breath. Some did have shortness of breath but were ignored or dismissed due to medical racism, sexism, other biases, or an overwhelmed emergency response system. Other COVID long-haulers were not hospitalized in their acute phase, because their initial cases were mild, moderate, or even asymptomatic.

After two days in the hospital receiving supplemental oxygen, I was discharged. My oxygen levels had improved, and my fever had broken. The doctors treating me said I'd only need to return if those two symptoms worsened. As I waited to be discharged, I tried not to think about what I would do if those symptoms returned. I came as close to praying as this agnostic Jew ever has. The hospital was beginning to flood with patients, no visitors were allowed, and I wanted so badly to go home and stay there.

When I returned home that night, I felt a sweeping sense of relief. I'd made it. The hospital had been scary, but I would be all right. I had not died, like the young doctor in Wuhan whose story had appeared in the news the night I was admitted. My breathing, while still slightly labored, had not deteriorated. I cried with gratitude as I stumbled into my bedroom, still scattered with thermometers, Tylenol bottles, and the notebooks I'd been using to communicate when my shortness of breath was so severe that I couldn't speak. I was so relieved to be back. I'd stay confined in that room alone for the next two weeks to avoid infecting others, per my doctor's orders.

It took a few days for me to fully notice the new symptoms. I was grateful to be able to breathe, and so exhausted from my acute infection and hospitalization, that I didn't pay much attention to the loss of smell, distorted taste, or new post-nasal drip and sinus pain. But, when it became clear that I also couldn't properly digest any food, I started to worry. I'd stepped on a scale the day I was discharged and saw a number I hadn't seen since I was fourteen. I felt weak, and I was terrified that I'd only get weaker if I couldn't eat.

But the nurse at the hospital had said that gastrointestinal issues weren't a COVID symptom, and even though I'd vomited once in my acute phase and was experiencing daily bouts of debilitating diarrhea after every attempt to eat, I wanted to trust the medical advice I'd been given. Plus, I'd sought other opinions. I'd googled the Centers for Disease Control's symptom list, which only included respiratory symptoms and fever. I'd emailed my PCP to ask if the GI symptoms could be connected to my COVID infection; she didn't know. I began to develop a new theory: My sudden and increasing nasal congestion and sore throat were due to early spring allergies, and my GI issues were food poisoning from meals I'd barely eaten at the hospital. The extreme fatigue, headaches, and sinus pain? A product of all three, I figured. But when I started to break out in hives and rashes, I was no longer able to explain away what was happening.

Part II: Finding My Person

During those first two weeks of illness, Sabrina and I kept in touch as best we could, but it was hard. I could barely find the energy to email my doctor or update my parents via text. I deleted Instagram, Twitter, and every news app, because I knew I needed to remain calm to maximize the little oxygen I had. The news—all about coronavirus—was terrifying and anxiety-producing. After I tested positive, I'd posted an alert on Instagram and contacted people who I might have infected, but my conversations about my illness had still mainly been limited to health care workers.

Sabrina had similarly been struggling to manage her care and learn about this illness. I had provided her with the first step: my own positive COVID test result would allow her to better confirm her own case. At the time, tests and clinical diagnoses were generally being reserved for hospitalized patients, people who had traveled to certain international locations, and those with a confirmed close contact. Sabrina now had a confirmed close contact (though the rules for who could test would continue to change). In return, she told me what she'd learned on social media and asked me questions: "Was I having trouble with smell and taste? Did I feel like I had a stomach flu?" She showed me a Twitter thread from an actor who said she'd lost her sense of smell, and together we found a small news article about a Princess Cruises passenger with GI symptoms.

By late March, I had managed to write a short op-ed in *The New York Times* about my experience being hospitalized with COVID as a twenty-six-year-old and had received messages on social media from other young COVID patients around the world. I told Sabrina that some of these people had cases that sounded similar to hers: no severe shortness of breath, but significant multi-systemic symptoms, including low-grade fevers that had lasted for weeks. The more Sabrina and I talked and shared our experiences, the more we realized how little information there was for people like us. News coverage at the time almost seemed to completely ignore the human experience of battling the disease. We felt totally alone. We *were* totally alone.

At the same time, my conversations with Sabrina (all via text and FaceTime) had broken the seal on my bubble of isolation. Hearing about her symptoms and sleuthing for answers together made me feel—for the first time since I'd gotten sick—completely understood and a tiny bit more in control of my own destiny.

When you're struggling alone, desperate for information, all you really need is one person who understands and believes you. It's pretty rad if this person also happens to share childhood memories of Hell's Kitchen, tells great feminist jokes, and is one of your best friends, but, as I've learned, you don't actually need to have much in common with another long-hauler to find mutual understanding and comfort. Over the past two years, I've developed friendships with people who are very different from me—a parent in Chicago, an artist in the United Kingdom, and an academic in South Africa, to name a few—all through the lens of our shared experiences with Long COVID.

Sabrina and I knew what we had in those conversations and texts, and that it was special. We wanted other patients to have that experience, too. So, on March 26, we launched a COVID support group through Body Politic. The rest is, well, history.

Part III: Who Is an Expert on Long COVID?

If you've ever had a serious illness or have cared for someone with a serious illness, you may be aware that there's a range of people who see pain, fear, and sickness and attempt to provide answers. Some of these people are medical professionals, trying to do their job. Others are well-meaning health or wellness enthusiasts. Some are just out to capitalize on your experience or scam you. Not all advice is created equal.

When Sabrina and I got sick, there were no COVID experts. I now know that there were people with post-viral and infection-initiated chronic illnesses, like myalgic encephalomyelitis (once called chronic fatigue syndrome and often abbreviated as ME/CFS), who knew that the pandemic would likely result in a mass-disabling event and who could speak to the experience of living with a complex, multi-systemic, chronic illness. These people, and the providers and researchers who have worked with them, would eventually become a source of vital information (you'll read more about them in this book). But, back in March of 2020, all that I knew was that no one—not the doctors treating me, not the international or federal health agencies, not even the infectious disease experts talking on CNN—could explain what was happening to my body. I could keep waiting around for them to find answers (or, at the very least, acknowledge my pain), or I could learn from others who have been neglected or ignored by medicine and science, and crowdsource the information myself. I wasn't a scientist—hell, I'd been a history major. But it turned out that history degree would come in handy.

As soon as I had enough energy to open my laptop, I started digging around for old college syllabi, rereading first-person accounts of the AIDS Coalition to Unleash Power (ACT UP) and other activist groups that provided peer-to-peer support, care, and knowledge-gathering during the HIV/AIDS epidemic. I reread a book about people who taught themselves how to perform abortions before they were legal and paged through old photos of medical clinics run by the Black Panthers. I'd analyzed all these texts in school, but reading them felt different this time. A common theme was emerging: If you think no one cares about you, you might be right . . . and you might need to do it yourself.

This book is authored primarily by people who have experienced Long COVID; most are still living with the illness. Their professional and personal backgrounds are diverse, some have degrees in science or medicine, others are professional writers, educators, or activists, but their most important qualification is their lived experience. Having reported closely on Long COVID since it first emerged, I can tell you firsthand that it was the actions of long-haulers themselves that triggered a global response to this illness. Nearly every piece of knowledge we have gained about this disease, as well as every attempt to provide systemic support, would not exist without the leadership and input of Long COVID patients. We are the reason it has a name, a disease classification code, interim guidance, dedicated clinics, a page on the CDC website,[1] and funded research. Obviously, there are also a lot of allies outside of our lived experience, journalists, scientists, and medical professionals, to name a few, who have raised awareness and carefully listened to our stories, using them to inform scientific research and sometimes making major breakthroughs (you'll hear from a couple of these people in this book). We wouldn't be where we are today without them. But a guidebook on Long COVID must be authored by those who have experienced it firsthand—and ideally a diverse group, given the varying disease presentations and experiences that can characterize this illness. Otherwise, we are rewriting history, plagiarizing ideas, and—honestly—likely to get a lot wrong.

That's because patients have been able to learn about Long COVID for longer, and from a much more intimate vantage point, than anyone else.

From day one in the support group, I was learning. I learned that hives and rashes were not unusual and that many long-haulers were experiencing histamine or allergic reactions to triggers that were either previously unknown or had proved harmless in the past. I learned that GI symptoms were also common and that some patients were unable to leave their bathrooms for days. I learned that the painful headaches that made my eyes burn and forced me to turn off all light or sound stimuli were likely migraines. I learned that when my body ached for rest, that was exactly what I should give it. I learned from people experiencing symptoms for the first time and from people with years of experience managing chronic illnesses. We learned together.

Remember when I said that all you need is one person who truly understands what you're going through and believes you? For me, that person was Sabrina. Then, it was ten thousand strangers on the internet. Today, it is a wide network that includes providers, health experts, disability justice advocates, and friends and family. You may not be fortunate to have such a network yet, and that's common. Long COVID is still widely misunderstood. I hope this book can be the start of such a network for you. I hope it envelopes you in a warm hug of words that resonate with your experience and promises you that, at bare minimum, you are believed, your life matters, and you certainly are not alone.

Part IV: A Few Things to Keep in Mind . . .

Notes About Language

This book contains a glossary on page 257, filled with medical and scientific terms related to Long COVID and navigating health care and disability benefits systems. Each chapter will also attempt to explain these terms within the context of that chapter's theme. But I want to share a few definitions of my own here that you may not find elsewhere.

Healing and Recovery: The words *healing* and *recovery* may appear from time to time in this book and are defined loosely throughout. While some Long COVID patients may make partial or full physical recoveries from their illness, most of our authors are not referring to full physical recoveries when they use this term.

For most of us, the experience of contracting and managing Long COVID has been a journey—one often peppered with traumatic experiences, pain, and loss. When we write about the journey to recovery or healing, we are generally referring to a process that may include better understanding one's illness, accessing better medical care or caregiving, processing traumas in a safe environment, rebuilding a (potentially new) sense of self and identity, connecting with community, and finding moments of joy again. If you've been expecting to make a full physical recovery, you may feel disappointed reading my definition of healing, but please know that many of these seemingly small improvements to quality of life can, in fact, be lifesaving.

Lastly, as someone who did experience significant improvement in my Long COVID symptoms, I can tell you that there is much more to healing than just physical recovery. I am not the person I was before I developed Long COVID, and I doubt I will ever feel I've returned to that former self, even if all of my remaining health issues someday evaporate. Like many of the contributors in this book, I feel changed by what I have witnessed—not just in my own body, but in those who got sick with me, in those who turned away from our pain, and in all those who mobilized on our behalf. There are losses to be grieved, and there are also new selves to be acknowledged—and, in some cases, celebrated.

Care: The term *care* is used throughout this book to mean several different things. In some cases, *care* refers to *medical care* provided by a licensed health care professional. In other cases, *care* refers to the generalized concept of support, which may come from fellow long-haulers, family and friends, employers, or medical professionals. The term *care* is also deeply tied to the *caring economy* and caregivers; many long-haulers receive the majority of their care at home. As I have learned from caregiving experts like Raj and Anjali Mehta, care in caregiving relationships is often multi-directional. Sometimes that sort of care will be referenced in this book—care that ties communities or networks together, taking many forms across multiple directions.

Long COVID and COVID-19 Long-Haulers: The term *Long COVID* typically refers to symptoms following a COVID-19 infection that last for more than four weeks. You'll read various clinical definitions of this illness in this book, some of which go into greater detail about common symptoms and ways to be diagnosed. It's important to touch on the origin of these terms. *Long COVID* and *COVID-19 long-hauler* (*"long-hauler"*) are both terms that were first coined by patients experiencing the disease. In May 2020, Italian academic Elisa Perego first tweeted "Long COVID" to describe her ongoing symptoms. A month earlier, Oregon-based preschool teacher Amy Watson joked that she was a "long-hauler," wearing a trucker-style baseball cap while she waited for a PCR test result for long-term COVID-19 symptoms.

Elisa and Amy gave us language for what we were going through before it was possible to receive a clinical diagnosis or even acknowledgment from most medical providers that COVID-19 could cause long-term symptoms. While both women prefer to emphasize the collective power of the patient community—I want to acknowledge them here. In naming our illness, they provided us with guiding lights for how to describe what we were going through and how to approach future advocacy. They made it clear that we patients wouldn't wait for science and medicine to acknowledge us; instead, we would move forward together—and everyone else would just have to catch up.

Disability: *Disability* is a term with a broad definition. During my journey with Long COVID, I learned about common misconceptions regarding who may identify as disabled. I'll debunk a few of those myths here:

1. Not all disabled people have visible physical disabilities. Many Long COVID patients, in particular, may read as non-disabled to people who are not aware of their illness. This doesn't mean they are not disabled. The term *invisible disability* is often used to describe such situations.

2. Some disabilities are permanent or long-lasting. Others, like a broken leg, may be temporary. Some people, like myself, like to identify as intermittently disabled, because our health issues wax and wane, causing us to experience disability at times, while at other times having the privileges of non-disabled people.

3. Not all people who use mobility aids, like wheelchairs, use them all the time, or identify as "wheelchair users." Some people use mobility aids as needed. Seeing someone with a wheelchair get up and walk is not proof that they are not disabled. Mobility aids can also be extremely helpful for people with episodic or intermittent health issues or disabilities; you will read recommendations about such aids in this book.

These are some general ideas to keep in mind as you read this book—and these notes only scratch the surface of misconceptions about disability—but ultimately people identify in different ways, using different terms. As a journalist, I generally take my cues from the people I'm interviewing, using the language they use to describe themselves. In this book, I've tried to do the same. I haven't changed anyone's language choices around the word *disability*, so you may see that term, and others, differ from chapter to chapter.

Relatedly, some folks in the disability community prefer identity-first language (e.g., *autistic person*) while others prefer person-first language (e.g., *person living with HIV*). I have connected more with the concept of identity-first language for myself, as I like the way it destigmatizes certain often-stigmatized terms by putting them front and center. That being said, everyone relates to these options differently. I haven't changed any of our authors' language around this either, so you will sometimes read person-first language and sometimes read identity-first language.

Similarly, different people relate differently to the term *patient*. I have liked the term *patient* for myself, but others feel it does not allow long-haulers to have an identity outside of their relationship to health care systems. As you can see, sometimes we use the term *long-hauler* on its own, instead of *patient*.

Setting Expectations: What This Book Is

During my Long COVID journey and my experience reporting and writing about the disease, it has become increasingly important to me to manage and set appropriate expectations. At the beginning of the first wave in the United States, many of us were told we would recover from COVID quickly (you will read this again and again in this book), and the dashing of those expectations caused me unnecessary additional pain. So, I want to be very clear with you now about what this book will and will not do.

This book will not

- promise recovery—full or partial
- provide one-size-fits-all advice
- promote a "cure-all" treatment plan (as one of this book's contributors David Putrino has often said, "Anyone who says they know how to cure Long COVID right now probably doesn't know anything at all or is trying to sell you something")
- push hero narratives, inspiration porn, or one person's story as the *right* way to navigate Long COVID.

This book will

- introduce you to a loving community of knowledgeable and supportive peers
- provide tips for emotionally healing from the traumatic experiences you may have had while contracting, dealing with, and pursuing care for a novel complex chronic illness
- offer logistical advice about financial hardship and workplace discrimination
- suggest symptom management advice for specific, common long-haul symptoms
- summarize crowdsourced guidance from health care professionals and patients on navigating health care systems
- explain current theories for Long COVID, existing research, and how to navigate the many research findings on this condition that will likely emerge in years to come

- offer guidance and acknowledge the very real ways racism, sexism, homophobia, fatphobia, ableism, capitalism, and other systems and forms of oppression may impact your quest for care and healing

- contextualize your experience within a larger history of neglected complex chronic illnesses and explain how this knowledge can be useful to you

- reassure you that no matter what you have been through, or how you may have been treated by others, you are not alone, and you are not forgotten.

Who Is and Who Isn't Left Out

A book on Long COVID cannot capture every patient's experience. To start, the umbrella of symptoms associated with Long COVID is too large to represent in one single book. The chapters in this book focus on some of the more common and widespread health issues and diagnoses (like fatigue, cognitive dysfunction or "brain fog," post-exertional symptom exacerbation, and dysautonomia) as well as overarching themes related to seeking care, managing relationships and finances, and navigating mental health issues.

Within Long COVID and related illnesses, there is also a spectrum of severity, and that spectrum is not entirely represented in this book. While our contributors have had diverse illness experiences and many have participated in this project in unique ways that fit their individual capacities, many of the people most marginalized by this disease are not included in this book. I say this because the most marginalized Long COVID patients are often those who have been disabled by this disease but do not know they have Long COVID, or who have been left without the time or ability to participate in a project like this. In some cases, Long COVID patients have died by suicide.

I want to take a moment here to honor the many people who have disappeared from society as a result of the many difficulties that exist in accessing the care and financial support necessary to survive—let alone contribute a chapter to a book. For those interested in learning more about this phenomenon, I recommend checking out the #MillionsMissing campaign that ME/CFS advocates created years ago to recognize all those in their community who are missed for similar reasons.

Who This Book Is For

You don't have to have Long COVID to read this book. In fact, I hope this book is read by many people who don't have the disease, because if prevalence estimates prove correct, it's likely we will all know someone with Long COVID eventually, and it's likely we will all have to step into a position of providing care, even in tiny ways, for those disabled by this pandemic. There are many insights in this book that are relevant for caregivers, providers, employers, and family members who may love, care for, or interact with COVID long-haulers.

This book also contains insights from chronic illness communities that predate the Long COVID patient community. In return, I hope this book provides some relatable stories and insights that are useful to other chronic illness communities. This is a book about Long COVID, and so it is also a book about the experience of being chronically ill in a society that generally fails chronically ill and disabled people. I think a lot of people can relate to that.

Finally, a word on support groups. Most of the contributors in this book met in the Body Politic support group, or one of the actions, initiatives, or communities that have stemmed from it. We have attempted to replicate the community, love, and support we've found there in these pages. But you don't need to be a fan or a member of a support group to read this book. If you find those groups overwhelming or difficult to access, I hope this book provides a helpful alternative. Also, it's worth mentioning that support groups come in many forms. The contributors to this book connected via social media because that was easiest when we were many miles away from one another and confined to our bedrooms. But you may find a support group of sorts in your coworkers, your family, your school, or your neighborhood. Despite what you may think, long-haulers and those who care for us are everywhere, and support could show up in a place you least expect it. I want to take a moment here to honor the many chronically ill people who have seemingly disappeared from society as a result of the difficulties that exist in accessing the care and financial support necessary to survive—let alone contribute a chapter to a book.

How This Book Relates to the
Future of Long COVID

The task of writing a guidebook to a novel chronic illness is not easy. There is so much we still don't know, and so much that will likely be revealed in years and decades to come (fingers crossed!). In this book, we spend slightly less time on current theories and experimental treatments, because we want the advice provided here to remain useful for years to come. We also recognize that many current new treatments are difficult to access, either because of financial barriers or because they haven't been approved everywhere. In placing more emphasis on tried-and-true symptom management techniques and social, emotional, and systems-related issues connected to Long COVID, I believe we have created a book that will be relevant for a long time and can support a diverse range of people grappling with complex chronic illnesses, new disabilities, and biased medical systems.

When I first embarked on this project, I believed I was writing for the existing cohort of Long COVID patients at the time. Then Delta hit, then Omicron, and so on. As a first-waver, I've stopped counting new waves. I only know there are more and more of us each day—crossing my Twitter feed with new questions or entering the support group with an introduction that often includes the phrase, "I thought I was alone until I joined this group." I hope beyond hope that the waves of Long COVID cease soon, but *just in case*, I'm prepared for the idea that we are unlikely to eradicate viruses, post-viral disease, complex chronic illness, or pandemics in my lifetime. If anything, I expect to see more of this as I age.

I hope this book provides insights to those who may come after us. I hope that it provides a model for future patient-to-patient and peer-to-peer support. I hope that maybe someday it serves as a historical artifact—proof that we were here and that we cared for one another. Most of all, I hope that on a dark or difficult day it provides what I needed most on my dark and difficult days: a place you can turn to for unequivocal support, understanding, and validation.

CHAPTER 1

It Wasn't the Beans and Rice

Fighting Biased Health Care Systems with Community Care

Karla Monterroso

O n my fifty-third day of COVID symptoms, I felt incredibly faint. My chest hurt in a way I had only heard about in public health leaflets about women's heart attacks. I had been to urgent care and the hospital twice since March 13, 2020, and all of the health care providers had been so disinterested that I had no faith that returning would result in anything useful. During every previous visit, doctors had questioned whether my symptoms were a result of my weight. I am a plus-size Latina and a weightlifter; before COVID, I could deadlift 220 pounds. Yet whenever I stepped into a medical facility, the first thing most doctors talked about was my size, often making assumptions about my eating habits and Mexican food.

According to them, it was my weight and the foods my family had been eating for generations that were causing my shortness of breath while laying down, tachycardia every time I stood or emoted, the feeling of an elephant sitting on my chest, and the random shocks of pain in my calves, in my abdomen, and underneath my fingernails. No matter how fit I was, my weight and ethnicity were always at fault for every malady I sought care for from health providers. That had been the case my whole adult life, so I was used to spending months researching and looking for doctors who would treat me as whole and human whenever I needed care. But it's impossible to do that kind of research in a medical emergency, especially one spurred by a pandemic, and especially when you're sick with something that has you sleeping for sixteen hours a day.

So on that morning of my fifty-third day of COVID illness, when I understood that my symptoms were very serious and that health care providers were unlikely to treat them as such, I did the first thing that came to mind, and called in sick to work. I wanted to prepare my coworker for the idea that I might never return to work; I might not make it through this at all. "It's perfectly possible that I don't make it to tomorrow," I said over the phone to Mimi Fox Melton, the general manager at the nonprofit where I was CEO. "If I don't, here are the instructions for the organization."

Mimi later told me my tone on that call was oddly matter-of-fact. By that point in my illness, I had gone numb and was over-functioning to avoid the anxiety, rage, and utter fear that thinking about being this sick—with no recourse— would trigger. I believed my illness was too far gone, and that the overwhelmed health care system would let me die. I fluctuated between trying to survive and preparing the people around me that I might not. Mimi, chilled by what she had heard in my voice, told me she'd call me back and hung up, because she needed to release her own terrified emotions before trying to support me. Meanwhile, I laid on the couch trying to catch my breath. I was having trouble breathing, my heart rate was incredibly high, and I couldn't stop feeling dizzy—especially when I stood up.

Luckily, my coworkers and my family weren't emotionally numb like I'd become, and they were not willing to give up on me. When Mimi called me back ten minutes later she said, "I want you to pack up and go to the hospital." *Please don't make me*, I thought. My past experiences at the hospital had made me feel so unsafe in a place where you should feel safest. I didn't say this to Mimi. Instead, like a person who has been to a lot of therapy, I asked her to help me understand why she thought that was a good idea.

"Karla, you just fucking told me you think you're going to die," she said, "I need you to go to a place where that won't happen." She told me she'd called her cousin, Jacinda, who was a cardiac nurse; Jacinda had recommended I go to the hospital immediately.

I was scared. "They don't see me there," I said.

"I know," she said, "but here's what you're going to do: Put on some minimal makeup. Make yourself as 'presentable human' as possible, and then go down there and make them treat you like a human."

I didn't feel I had the energy to make myself presentable, advocate for myself, or go back to that horrible place. But Mimi told me she and Jacinda would FaceTime with me the whole time, since they couldn't come in person (visitors weren't allowed in the ER). Still, I wasn't sure. I needed another perspective.

I proceeded to make phone calls to my brother and two of my best friends. I asked each of them the same question: "Here are my symptoms, do *you* think I need to go to the hospital?" Everyone agreed I should go.

"It's okay, Karla," my brother said, "We've entered the 'too scary to handle on your own' phase." I thought, but didn't say, *I feel like I've been in the "too scary to handle on my own" phase since the fourth day of symptoms*. But I knew he was right. Armed with my cell phone, charger, and the knowledge that Mimi and Jacinda would be my health care advocates via FaceTime, I called the ambulance.

On day fifty-three of fevers, difficulty breathing, no smell or taste, crippling pain, headaches, chest aches, cycling oxygen levels, vomiting, and feeling like my body was on fire, I stood at my bedroom mirror and put on makeup so a hospital would treat me like a human.

I was soon met with an ambulance and EMTs who measured my blood pressure, which was 75/52 (my normal blood pressure is usually around 118/77). The EMTs ran the test three times, not believing the numbers. It took so long that a neighbor, who was watching from a distance, yelled at them to put me in the ambulance and retest there.

I arrived at the hospital and the physician came in ready to discharge me before even conducting an exam. He said COVID doesn't exist in the body for fifty-three days; there was no way I could still be sick. When Mimi and Jacinda (a cardiac nurse!) asked questions and pushed back on FaceTime, the doctor went ballistic. He refused to treat me while they were on the phone. I could get health care *only* if my advocates weren't present.

I was woozy and having a very hard time communicating. Yet I wasn't allowed to have help. When the doctor came back, he brought up my friends and my "tone." I told him I needed him to focus on my health care, not our attitudes. While I was struggling to put my words together due to my cognitive symptoms, the doctor derisively asked if I spoke Spanish. He then asked multiple times if my symptoms were diabetes related. I had never been even prediabetic.

Meanwhile, I knew my oxygen levels needed to be at 95 or higher to be considered normal and, at that moment, they were cycling from the 70s to the low 90s. But the doctor told me the 70s didn't count and that I shouldn't worry about it—it probably meant that I was cold. If the reading were true, he said, I would be out of breath. It was May of 2020, and I had already seen articles about "happy hypoxia," a phenomenon where COVID patients present with low oxygen saturation levels but do not appear to be struggling to breathe. I had the articles pulled up on my phone and I tried to tell the doctor about them, but he grew insulted.

As a weightlifter, I was acutely aware of how my body behaved. According to my Apple Watch, my pre-COVID resting heart rate was 65. But, laying in that hospital bed, my heart rate stayed above 130 for at least five hours; if I sat up, it would rocket into the 150s. At its peak, my tachycardia was up to 188. *How long can a heart beat at that rate before it causes serious issues*, I wondered.

Meanwhile my friends—a community of activists, lawyers, and leaders of color—were taking my stats to doctors of color who they knew. They wanted to see if we were right to be concerned about my condition or if the care I was receiving was annoying, but accurate. Three doctors confirmed that I should at least be getting IV liquids and that I should be admitted to the hospital overnight for my accelerated heart rate alone. As I calmly but firmly discussed this with the attending physician, he again became irate, telling me how inappropriate it was to seek outside information. He asked for the other doctors' numbers, so he could tell them how unprofessional they were. I said I wanted a different doctor, and he told me there were no other doctors. I said I wanted a patient advocate, and he said they might be able to connect me with someone in the morning.

I am among the top 10 percent of wage earners in the Latinx community. I was an executive. I had previously worked in health care and knew what I could ask for. I had a large and well-connected community. Even then, every resource I tried to access through the hospital was denied to me.

I've thought back to many parts of that day, and the detail that always undoes me is that, although I was sick enough to need emergency health care, I first paused to put on decent clothes and makeup. I did it in the vain hope that it would change the course of my care.

Women of color are unsafe in our health care system—we are not believed and often treated with suspicion. Health care providers tell us that our health issues are our own making or a figment of our imagination. A 2020 study from the JAMA Network tells us that one in five patients have faced discrimination of some kind in a health care setting. Of those who faced discrimination, 72 percent experienced it more than once.[1] But we are still asked, at the most vulnerable and scary moments of our lives, to turn to those institutions for help.

During this pandemic, the death rate for Black and Latinx people has been two times that for their white peers.[2] The media has ascribed this discrepancy in death rates to similar discrepancies in comorbidities, driven by a vast racial wealth gap. While this is true—and profoundly unjust for our communities—this explanation alone discounts a large part of the experience of Asian, Native, and Black and/or non-Black Latinx people seeking care. We are also dying because we are being sent home over and over again, until our conditions are too severe to be treated effectively. We are dying because we're often treated as invisible, and when we demand visibility, we are viewed as insubordinate.

Long COVID presents in many, many, many different forms, but common symptoms are fatigue that makes you feel like weights have been strapped to your shoulders, chest, abdomen, and legs—demanding that you stay in bed; brain fog that makes you feel like your brain has to travel through a soupy marsh to articulate a single thought; a limited supply of energy that gets depleted by walking or thinking too much; and the constant feeling of being out of breath. Coincidentally, stereotypes about Latinx, non-Latinx Black, and Native people are that we're lazy, stupid, and have unhealthy diets. So, what do you do when the disease you have contracted presents as the very stereotypes people believe about you and your community?

Having lost all faith in the physician and the hospital I visited that day, I left "AMA," against medical advice. When I told the physician I was leaving, he told me I could have a heart attack between this hospital and the next place I sought care. Suddenly, my condition was serious to him. With great effort, I got up and tried to close the door to start putting my clothes on. He wouldn't let me, placing his body in the doorway: "You're risking your life if you leave," he said. "If you stay, we might admit you."

"I need you to understand that I absolutely know that is a possibility," I said. "But I have lost so much faith in you and this hospital that I believe staying here would be a bigger risk to my life. Please let me close this door."

With the door shut, I proceeded to dress myself, moving as slowly as possible to minimize the discomfort. Through the door, the doctor continued to yell, insisting that I give him the names and phone numbers of the other medical professionals I had accessed so he could talk to their managers. I leaned on the door and waited for his voice to fade. Finally, I walked as fast as my heart could muster to the parking lot where a friend in full PPE was waiting to take me to another hospital.

I had tried to keep many of my symptoms private, only divulging how serious my illness was to a small circle of people I trusted completely, so as not to worry too many people. But once Mimi witnessed my experience at the ER, she began employing a network of friends and colleagues to save me. In the end, it was a friend in New York who came through, calling in a favor at UCSF hospital where she knew people. While I was arguing with the doctor at the first hospital, UCSF was preparing for my arrival. Once there, I was admitted within an hour and hooked up to IV fluids quickly. The staff would go on to treat me with care.

I have always been an overachiever. I am the kind of person who actively works to "handle" the emergencies that pop up. For the first six months of my illness, two cardiologists, a rheumatologist, and a primary care provider encouraged me to push through my fatigue, to exercise, and to resume normal activity. I was told I just needed to recondition my body to activity.

I would call doctors and tell them about the impacts of doing just that. I would report that "pushing through" was increasing my pain and tachycardia and sending me to bed for weeks on end. I had fallen in the shower on five different occasions after getting woozy when the tachycardia would hit its peak. At the same time, the ME/CFS community was warning anyone who would listen that the country was about to be hit with millions of people whose post-viral conditions would require deep rest for at least six weeks to prevent further disablement. My doctors' advice to exercise and push through symptoms was in direct opposition to these disabled folks' wisdom. I wish I had found them first.

I know now that some of the decisions I made in those first months prolonged my condition. I try hard not to blame myself; I thought I was doing the right thing by following every piece of medical advice I received. I remember describing to my first cardiologist—a white man—the crashes in energy and ability that would follow after I pushed myself to my limit. He responded, "Sometimes we just don't want to get back to it. It's nice staying in bed. But you need to get up. Entiende?"

I've often tried to explain away this bad advice, telling myself that in the spring and summer of 2020 we were in the early stages of a pandemic, and no one understood Long COVID. There were no good answers. There were no treatments. When I think back to this time, I also remember that first cardiologist with his condescending "Entiende?" and the burning feeling of embarrassment on my face as he inferred that my inability to "be better" was a product of my own laziness.

It was irresponsible for doctors to be so confident about a disease that we are still learning about. I knew in my body that their advice was wrong, but I felt I had no choice but to trust them and their experience over my own intuition. I will not be doing that again.

Throughout my life, I've had to grapple with a relationship to productivity that is unique to people of color. We understand that this country will reject us if we stop "contributing." My job, which allowed for medical leave, provided me with a lot of privileges. I kept trying to do things because I felt a sense of guilt around that fear of "laziness." The value of hard work has been drilled into me since I was a toddler. My mother is from Mexico and my father is from Guatemala; both of them innately understood that my ability to work hard was critical to my value growing up in the United States. This is a message that is reaffirmed in the media. There are "good" people of color and "bad" people of color—and you do not want to be one of the bad ones.

While there is nothing wrong with being a hard worker, my attachment to the concept drove me to develop a lot of terrible tendencies. In fact, I have spent my entire adult life trying to understand how those perceptions have impacted my tendency to work compulsively. In this country, 20 percent of Latinx people aged twenty-five and older have a bachelor's degree or higher, and 10.4 percent of Latinx people are in management or professional industries.[3] We are overrepresented in low-wage jobs and underrepresented in high-wage jobs. Our hold in salaried work is tenuous, and any indication that you may not work "twice as hard," as the old adage goes, is a reason to take away your livelihood.

A 2016 study by the Public Religion Research Institute revealed that 75 percent of white people have all-white social networks, 16 percent have one person of color in their close social networks, and only 9 percent have a diversity of people in their social networks.[4] This means that most people in high-wage work only come into contact with Latinx people working low-wage service jobs and through the depictions they see in the media. This is a plight shared by non-Latinx Black and Native people as well. The USC Annenberg Inclusion Initiative cites that only 5 percent of all characters in films are Latinx, and 40 percent of the top billed Latinx characters depicted are violent criminals.[5] It's more likely for a mid- to high-wage white American to consume media representing Latinx people as criminals than it is for them to come into contact with a salaried Latinx professional.

Meanwhile, we do nothing to recognize the value in those who perform low-wage work. Even the language that we often use to describe this work—"unskilled"—underplays the tremendous level of skill being performed every day by people in professions the economy constantly devalues; people doing farm work, child and elderly care work, and food service work are skilled yet unprotected workers. For a brief moment, we called these people essential workers—and then quickly made decision after decision that put them in precarious positions where they had to choose whether to expose themselves and their families to this virus or lose their jobs. It's hard to describe what that precarity does to you, especially when you grew up in a working-class household and are the first in your family to know the stability of salaried work. People of color are constantly making trade-offs, deciding whether to prioritize their financial stability over their health and well-being. When this pandemic hit, we were made to feel like we were heroes for making that trade-off—as long as we kept making it.

There were two game-changing moments in my experience. The first was finding an infectious disease specialist and woman of color who was recommended by my puzzled primary care provider. Dr. Yenjean Hwang was excellent. The first time I sat with her and told her my symptoms, she responded immediately, "You're not the only one. There are many of you. I don't know all the answers—we're figuring out this disease every day—but we're going to work on finding them together." She was the first specialist to acknowledge that what I was going through was more than a personal motivation problem. I cried tears of relief on and off for four hours after that appointment.

Again, I am in the top 10 percent of income earners in my Latinx community. My health insurance at the time was a PPO, which meant that I could choose from a large slate of specialists and visit those specialists without a referral from a primary care provider. Many people in my community do not have the same access—they aren't even allowed to see specialists if the first doctor they see doesn't believe their symptoms, which is not uncommon. I grieve for those folks and what our health care system has done to them.

The face of Long COVID in popular conversation has been primarily white. We aren't hearing the voices of Black, Latinx, Native, or Asian long-haulers. This isn't a coincidence. How many undiagnosed long-haulers are out there being gaslit by their medical providers because of the bias we *know* is happening in the medical community? How many long-haulers are being forced back into work before their bodies have healed, giving them even longer-term or more severe disabilities? Sometimes I question how public I've been about such a private and vulnerable medical situation. When I have these doubts, I think of those people, the folks without large platforms or resources like mine, who keep being told this is all in their heads because their providers believe they're exaggerating or trying to "get away" with an extended medical leave.

The second game-changing moment in my experience was when my colleague Mimi pulled the need for productivity out of my hands. I had been trying so hard to lead my organization after my most severe phase of COVID. But after the hospital visits she'd helped facilitate, she called me up and told me I was no longer going to be working. My short-term sick leave was now a long-term medical leave. We both knew I was struggling too much and not doing my organization or myself any good. Mimi told me I needed rest, real rest. After Mimi told me she had my duties covered, and that taking care of my job was no longer on the list of things I had to do, I slept for sixteen hours straight.

It was after that moment that my real journey to healing began. My whole focus became sleep, other kinds of rest, hydration, slow and steady physical rehabilitation with a qualified physical therapist who understood my limits, and a variety of medication regimens. I let myself be bored for the first time in my adult life. I read when I could focus enough to read. Mostly, I wrapped myself in the love of the people around me. At thirty-nine years old, I moved in with my parents six days out of the week. I took six months to transition back to life on my own.

My efforts to get healthy happened in the background while my whole world was being severely impacted by this disease. Over the course of the pandemic, I've had thirty-seven friends and family members get sick. Seventeen loved ones have ended up in the hospital. Two have died. It was like I got hit by a train, then had to scream warnings from the train tracks because I couldn't yet get myself up from them. I was often the first person people came to with questions, because I'd been one of the first to get sick. So, I created an onboarding guide to do the emotional labor that I was no longer able to do. This onboarding guide has been used by family, friends, and strangers alike. It has advice for the acute phase of the disease and what to do as you transition into being a long-hauler. You'll find an edited version of this guide on page 28.

According to Pew Research Center, 52 percent of Latinx people in the United States know someone who was either hospitalized or died from COVID. We account for 29 percent of COVID cases, even though we are only 18 percent of the population.[6] I felt those conditions in my multi-generational and multi-class family. When my grandmother passed away from COVID in December of 2020—her second bout with the disease—it took months before I felt her death as anything other than my failing her: failing to get to my family before disinformation, failing to help them understand the severity of my condition, and failing to ensure she was protected from a world very much in denial about COVID's repercussions.

There's a very weird tension between knowing that you were systematically failed by your country and knowing how lucky you were to escape with your life. For my medical, financial, and emotional needs, I found cheerleaders and systems in my community to help me. Even when I faced the mountains of challenges that are constant in the lives of people of color in America, there was an equal and opposing force trying to save me. I have family and friends who made every effort to ensure that I was fed, cared for, and defended. They had the resources to do so. I also know that I am an exception. Most people in my community don't have my luxuries. We are facing a disability crisis that is having and will continue to have a disproportionate impact on Latinx, and non-Latinx Black, and Native people, and there is no indication our country is preparing itself for this crisis.

We need to put governmental and nonprofit systems between people of color and the discrimination we're facing. In their absence, we need to set up community structures that support us. By creating these systems, we'd greatly increase the odds that *all* Long COVID patients get the resources and support they need. Yet, here we are, more than two years into this pandemic and not a single systemic intervention outside of vaccines has been made. The American project is poised, yet again, to send the message that our lives are disposable if they are not of use to the economy.

The writer and scholar bell hooks said the following about love: "The word 'love' is most often defined as a noun, yet all the more astute theorists of love acknowledge that we would all love better if we used it as a verb." She goes on to say, "To truly love we must learn various ingredients—care, affection, recognition, respect, commitment, and trust, as well as honest and open communication."[7]

I am forever altered by my illness experience. For all of the terrible things COVID did, it is with this definition of love in mind that I tell you that it taught me how to love and be loved. I was loved by my community in the truest sense. While it's heartbreaking to know we aren't loved in this way by our own country, I've watched with pride as we've used our collective power to ensure our mutual survival in a time of obscene trauma and illness. It is this love that has me sitting here, reflecting on these stories in service to what I hope is your acknowledgment, catharsis, care, and eventual healing. There's a version of me that could not have allowed herself to be helped in the way I've been helped because of the relationship to productivity and work that I held not very long ago. But we cannot do this alone. We need one another. So, whatever way it happens for you— with the people around you or people online—find your people. I'm clearer now than I've ever been: We are all we've got.

Survival Tips:
Karla's COVID Onboarding Guide

Medical Tools

Get a good infrared thermometer if you don't already have one. You will also want a pulse oximeter. It's good to take your oxygen levels, even for your own sanity. The second you are getting into the lower 90s (< 93), get in touch with a health care provider.

Diet

Dietary needs may fluctuate, depending on what cluster of symptoms you're experiencing, but as a general rule, try to make sure you are getting protein, iron, and electrolytes. Flood your system with Gatorade and broths. I was severely dehydrated every time I went to the hospital. Eventually, I got an electrolyte supplement with no sugar (Hydrus), but I recommend also drinking at least 120 ounces (3.5 L) of water a day. The inflammation really demands it.

Lots of folks are reporting vitamin D deficiencies, so I would stack myself with vitamin D. I also took vitamin C to bolster my immune system, and baby aspirin every morning, because COVID can thicken the blood and create blood clots. The second my fever got above 100°F (38°C), I would take Tylenol. I have now added the following vitamins to my Long COVID management: CoQ10 (for those who are tachycardic), B complex, zinc, omega-3, glutathione, and turmeric/ginger supplements. I have also added Tollovid, but it is prohibitively expensive for so many people and a sacrifice for me.

Managing Disease, Energy, and Comfort

Take naps on a schedule. It was helpful for me to picture this as a fight and think about how I could reinforce my body for it. You will feel so tired, for so long, that you will start to doubt yourself. You need a nap. Give your body a nap.

The congestion is crazy-making, because everything is inflamed but you also can't cough or blow your nose in the same ways. It's an everlasting leak. I steamed a lot, to give my body relief; it's about comfort as much as survival because, again, you're making your body a fighter. My doctor told me not to use a neti pot because of the risk of breathing in infected mucus.

Sleep propped up with pillows—lots of folks told me this, and I was skeptical. But the second I did it, I noticed my body wasn't struggling as much. It felt like I wasn't letting the virus settle in my chest.

Many have suggested sleeping prone (on your stomach). Laying in a prone position reduces pressure on the lungs and helps them expand fully. Your own personal comfort may determine which choice you make, but try to lay prone at least a few times a day.

The thing that worked best for me for the fever was getting on all fours in the shower with warm to cold water. This position let things drain out and helps congestion. If your fever and symptoms are lasting longer than two months, you likely have Long COVID and need to power down and rest.

Managing Mental Health

Long COVID is a yo-yo, and that's the most demoralizing part about it. One day you feel a little better, then the next day it slams you hard. It's not in your head; this is how it works. My prima, who is a COVID-19 investigator for San Diego County was like, "This thing is cruel. It wants you alone, it wants to give you hope and then crush it." So just be ready for the possibility of relief followed by a step backward.

COVID often makes you feel crazy—and the mental health battle is just as important. Be as kind as you can be to yourself. Yes, it's as scary as you think it is, but you are strong enough to beat it.

I made mantras for myself for the shower, morning, and night. You're going to battle, so you've got to help all the parts go to battle effectively.

Keeping Track

Keep a journal and monitor your temperature, heart rate, and breathing ability by the hour or every two hours. If you do need to be hospitalized, or even just see a health care provider, you'll be able to give that provider a lot of data.

Finding a Doctor

There will be a doctor out there who believes you. If your doctor doesn't currently believe you, there are many articles out there—I especially recommend the series Ed Yong did in *The Atlantic*—that discuss Long COVID. Bring your research with you. Information is power, and doctors don't know everything. If the doctor is quick to say it's in your head (which it's not), go find another doctor. I would especially recommend infectious disease specialists. If you can get a woman of color with experiences in communities of color, all the better. Working with communities of color is a competency. Don't undervalue that. If, for some reason, your insurance requires a referral to an infectious disease doctor from a primary care provider that doesn't believe you, demand that the primary care provider write in your chart that they denied the request and include the medical reasoning they are using to deny that care. This will allow you to make an appeal. Nine times out of ten, doctors do not want to make themselves liable in this way and will relent and give you a referral.

En Español

Herramientas

Obten un termómetro infrarojo si no lo tienes. También necesitas un pulsímetro para medir tu oxígeno. Es aconsejable tomar tu niveles de oxígeno. Inmediatamente notes que tu oxígeno baja en los 90s, llama a tu doctor.

Dieta

Es bueno comer comida alta en proteína, alto en hierro, tomar electrolitos. Toma suero, gatorade y caldos. Inmediatamente tu temperatura sube arriba de los 100 grados, toma Tylenol. Si tu temperatura no es muy alta, deja que tu sistema inmune pelee contra el virus. Alerta a la deshidratación, hay necesidad de tomar 120 onzas de agua con electrolitos por dia. La inflamación lo demanda.

Se ha reportado que mucha gente está deficiente de vitamina D, es bueno tomar cuando menos 800 mg. Al día, la vitamina C ayuda a reforzar el sistema inmune también. Es bueno tomar aspirina de bebe cada mañana porque COVID espesa la sangre y puede crear coágulos.

Manejando la enfermedad, la energía y la comodidad

Toma siestas regularmente. Es bueno para pelear la enfermedad y cómo reforzar tu cuerpo para pelearla. Te sentirás agotado continuamente. Necesitas siestas, dale siestas a tu cuerpo.

La congestión es desesperante haciéndote sentir todo tu sistema completamente inflamado, es difícil toser y sonar tu nariz regularmente, sientes la inflamación y controla totalmente tus vías respiratorias. Es aconsejable usar vaporizador, ayuda a relevar la incomodidad para respirar. Todo es tanto como la comodidad como la supervivencia. Estás haciendo de tu cuerpo un super peleador.

Es bueno dormir con varias almohadas para elevar tu cuerpo. Me aconsejaron hacerlo y lo dudé al principio, pero cuando lo empecé hacer, note la diferencia y mi cuerpo no batallaba tanto para respirar, sentí que de esta manera no dejaba que el virus se asentara en mi pecho.

Muchos han dicho que dormir o descansar boca abajo ayuda a reducir presión en tus pulmones y los deja expandir. Su preferencia personal la va guiar lo que escoje. Pero por lo menos has lo unos cuantos tiempos al dia.

Mi doctor me dijo que no usara Neti-pot porque hay riesgo que se aspire el moco infectado.

Una de las cosas que me ayudó para bajar la fiebre, fue el baño con agua tibia o al tiempo en mis manos y rodillas. La posición me ayudó a bajarla y también para la congestión.

Salud mental

Esta enfermedad es como un yo-yo, y también es una situación muy desmoralizante. Un día te sientes un poco mejor y al siguiente día te pega otra vez duro. Es bueno saber que no es solo en tu mente, esta es la manera en que esta enfermedad trabaja en los organizmos. En los hospitales mandan a la gente a casa y al regreso se ponen peor, precisamente porque es como una enfermedad yo-yo. Mi prima que es

Investigadora de COVID-19 en el condado de San Diego me dice que es lo cruel de esta enfermedad. Crees que te estas mejorando y después te das cuenta que estas igual de mal de regreso. Es Bueno te prepares tu mente para en caso te ocurra a ti.

La cosa que a veces lo descontrola mentalmente a uno es la pelea y es mejor prepararte mentalmente para esta pelea porque es tan importante como la recuperación de esta enfermedad.

Personalmente mi consejo es, fortalecerse mentalmente noche y día. Porque así como a mucha gente esta enfermedad no les hace mella, mucha gente muere y también a mucha gente—le pasa como a mi—lucha por meses para mejorarse y realmente es desesperante y desmoralizante.

Mantén un Diario escrito

Mantén un diario, toma tu temperatura y presión del corazón y la habilidad de respirar cada dos horas por lo menos. Para en caso que tengas que hablar con tu doctor o si necesitas hospitalización, tienes toda esta información a la mano.

Encontrar un médico

Habrá un médico que te crea. Si tu doctor/a no le cree, hay una serie de artículos que recomiendo—especialmente la serie que Ed Yong hizo en *The Atlantic*, que analiza Long Covid. Traiga sus materiales de investigación con usted. La información es poder y los médicos no lo saben todo. Si el médico le dice que la enfermedad está en su cabeza, no está en su cabeza, vaya a buscar otro médico. Recomiendo especialmente a un especialista en enfermedades infecciosas. Si puedes conseguir una mujer de color con experiencias en comunidades de color, mucho mejor. Trabajar con comunidades de color es una competencia. No subestimes esa competencia. Si por alguna razón su seguro médico requiere una recomendación de su médico primaria para ver un doctor de enfermedades infecciosas y el doctor primaria no quiere dárselo, dile al médico que escribe en su historial médico que le negó la solicitud y la razón médica que está usando para negar esa atención. Esto le permitirá presentar una apelación. Nueve de cada diez médicos no quieren hacerse responsables de esta manera y ceden y le darán una referencia.

CHAPTER 2

Standing Tall (and Sitting Right Back Down)

Living with Dysautonomia

Heather Hogan

I f you had asked me what was wrong with me two months after my initial COVID infection in March 2020, I would have sincerely told you, "Everything," and it wouldn't have been much of an exaggeration.

I got COVID during New York City's first wave, when tests, treatments, and even hospital space were nearly impossible to access. I had what was referred to as a "mild case," which meant I never needed to be put on a ventilator and that I'd survived. At the time, the guidelines for going to the hospital were: Don't do it unless you can't finish speaking a sentence out loud or your lips are turning blue. After about two weeks of a slight fever, shortness of breath, chest congestion, and moderate fatigue, I seemed to turn a corner and was well on my way back to my pre-COVID life, which included working sixty hours a week, volunteering, managing a full social calendar, riding my bike multiple times a week, and walking ten thousand steps every day. Despite the prevalence of post-viral illnesses prior to our pandemic, no provider, politician, or journalist had even mentioned the possibility of something like Long COVID. I thought I had beaten the "really bad flu."

Unfortunately, I didn't recover. Or, well, perhaps it's more accurate to say that while my body fought off the typical acute symptoms of COVID, I never returned to full health. In fact, I developed entirely new issues that hadn't been mentioned in the list of acute COVID symptoms: fatigue, an inability to regulate my body temperature, brain fog that caused me to forget simple words like *carrot*, erratic blood pressure, tachycardia, dizziness and near-fainting every time I stood up, new and more severe migraines, exercise intolerance, chest tightness, agitation, nausea and vomiting, and what seemed to be severe panic attacks at all hours of the day and night.

Over the course of several months, I saw my primary care physician multiple times, visited several urgent care doctors, and took a trip to the emergency room in an ambulance when I woke one night with blood pressure so high that the internet assured me I was having a stroke (I wasn't). The physical exams didn't reveal anything out of the ordinary. The bloodwork and scans my doctors ordered all came back normal. Over and over, I heard the same refrain from medical professionals: "It's just anxiety; the best thing you can do is get out in the sun and exercise."

I found myself sinking into a terrifying depression. I was unable to get out of bed for more than an hour or two a day, and even when I was out of bed, I wasn't able to do any of my pre-COVID activities, like working, exercising, socializing, or even unloading the dishwasher. Most days I couldn't keep my head up long enough to finish a full meal. I was waking up multiple times every night, drenched in sweat, with adrenaline coursing through my body. It was so extreme, my legs would move, mimicking the act of running (as if away from a bear attack!). I nearly passed out every time I moved from lying down to sitting or sitting to standing. My chest hurt, all lights were too bright, and I couldn't catch my breath—and yet, not a single doctor in New York City seemed to believe there was anything wrong with me.

My primary care physician suggested it was time to see a psychiatrist, and the psychiatrist agreed with the other doctors: Everything I was feeling was all in my head. Luckily, a friend who was experiencing similar post-COVID medical issues stumbled across an online support group where thousands of other people were experiencing symptoms like ours. It was there that I first heard of dysautonomia, from one of the very few doctors who was aware of what would become known as Long COVID, and from a support group moderator who'd developed dysautonomia from a viral infection years before.

Within a week I found a specialist who diagnosed me with postural orthostatic tachycardia syndrome (POTS), a type of dysautonomia.

What Is Dysautonomia?

Dysautonomia is a simple name for a complex group of medical conditions caused by dysregulation of the autonomic nervous system (ANS), the part of your nervous system that controls basically all the things your body does that you don't really think about or consciously make a decision to do: breathing, digestion, heart rate, blood pressure, body temperature, sleep cycles, bladder function, hormonal function, and more.

Dysautonomia can lead to a lengthy and diverse group of symptoms,[1] including

- blood pooling in extremities
- blurred vision or other visual disturbances
- brain fog and other cognitive impairment
- chest pain
- fainting
- fatigue
- gastrointestinal issues
- heart palpitations, tachycardia, bradycardia
- high or low or wildly fluctuating blood pressure
- inability to regulate body temperature, excessive sweating, no sweating
- low blood sugar
- migraines
- mood swings
- orthostatic intolerance (the inability to be upright without feeling dizziness, lightheadedness, vertigo)
- shaking
- shortness of breath.

Causes and Types of Dysautonomia

Prior to COVID, Dysautonomia International,[2] the leading nonprofit research and advocacy group for people with dysautonomia, estimated that the condition affected over seventy million people worldwide. That number will likely skyrocket in the coming years, owing to COVID and potential future pandemics. Dysautonomia can occur as its own disorder, or it can be secondary to other diseases, such as diabetes, Parkinson's disease, Sjogren's syndrome, Crohn's disease, celiac disease, and Ehlers-Danlos syndrome. It has commonly been diagnosed as a post-viral condition caused by hepatitis C virus, HIV, Epstein-Barr virus, influenza, and now COVID.

Because dysautonomia affects so many different organs and systems, there are, of course, many types of the disorder. Two of the most common types of adult-onset dysautonomia are

Neurally Mediated Hypotension (NMH),[3] which occurs when the ANS has trouble regulating blood pressure, especially when a person is upright. NMH is usually characterized by a drop in systolic blood pressure of 25 mm Hg or more and often leads to fainting, near-fainting, or tachycardia.

Postural Orthostatic Tachycardia Syndrome (POTS),[4] which occurs when the ANS has trouble regulating heart rate. People with POTS experience an increase in heart rate of 30+ BPM within ten minutes of standing (as opposed to an increase of 10 to 15 BPM, which occurs when a person without POTS stands up). POTS is also present if a person's heart rate reaches 120 BPM simply from standing, within ten minutes of standing.

These two types of dysautonomia are not mutually exclusive and are often diagnosed together. The thing they have in common, of course, is that issues often arise when a person is upright. When a person without dysautonomia sits or stands up, adrenaline causes the heart to beat just a little bit faster and with more force, causing blood vessels to constrict. This means that only a small amount of blood pools in the abdomen and lower body, and the rest finds its way back to the heart and to the brain without issue. In people with orthostatic intolerance (OI), that same system kicks in, but it doesn't work properly. Researchers don't fully understand why, but it appears that blood vessels in people with OI either don't constrict, or they dilate, which means more blood pools, less blood gets to the brain, the heart beats faster or blood pressure drops, and adrenaline keeps getting released. You can see why people with OI often experience lightheadedness, brain fog, heart issues, and fatigue.

Being upright is not the only trigger for people with dysautonomia. Being in a hot environment like the shower or a crowded street in the summer, experiencing emotional distress or stressful events, exercising, and even eating can exacerbate of symptoms due to blood pooling, redirected blood flow, and the release of too much epinephrine and norepinephrine (aka adrenaline).

Getting Diagnosed with Dysautonomia

When I arrived for my first appointment with the cardiologist who diagnosed me with POTS, she was surprised to see me. Not because she was shocked to learn that COVID had left me with dysautonomia—she was expecting an influx of new cases based on the many, many post-viral patients she'd diagnosed and treated over the years—but because I'd found her so quickly. It'd been months since I'd had COVID, and the bed-bound days and sleepless nights had felt like an eternity to me, but my cardiologist told me it often takes years for people who suffer with POTS to get properly diagnosed.

The reasons are myriad. There is, of course, the fact that the symptoms caused by dysautonomia aren't exclusive to dysautonomia so, more often than not, health care providers run tests on the more common—and life-threatening—potential reasons for the symptoms. When the bloodwork and imaging results come back clear, repeatedly, doctors often write off patients as having anxiety. A kind of confirmation bias often occurs in these situations, because autonomic dysfunction can mimic symptoms of anxiety disorder and panic disorder.

The autonomic nervous system is made up of two parts: the sympathetic nervous system (SNS) and the parasympathetic nervous system (PNS). The sympathetic nervous system is primarily responsible for the body's fight-or-flight response; it's the thing that revs up when it senses stress or danger, sending out a flood of hormones to boost the body's alertness and heart rate, making sure your muscles have enough blood, your brain has enough oxygen, and your blood has enough glucose to handle whatever threat it deems imminent. The parasympathetic nervous system works in tandem with the sympathetic nervous system. Once our bodies decide a threat has passed, our parasympathetic nervous system kicks in to return our body to homeostasis, bringing our breathing back to normal, lowering our blood pressure and heart rate, returning our hormones to their normal levels, and allowing us to get back to the "rest and digest" state.

Dysautonomia doesn't just cause dysfunction in the body parts it controls—heart, intestines, sweat glands, bladder, pupils, and blood vessels—it also causes trouble with communication between the parasympathetic nervous system and sympathetic nervous system, often leaving patients with their sympathetic nervous system "locked on," or in a lengthy state of fight-or-flight. This frequently results in what people with dysautonomia commonly refer to as "adrenaline dumps" or "adrenaline surges." Unfortunately, this is exactly the opposite of what happens in people with anxiety disorder or panic disorder. It's not anxiety manifesting as physical symptoms; it's physical symptoms manifesting in ways that look like anxiety.

My cardiologist also told me that people have a hard time getting diagnosed with dysautonomia because most dysautonomia patients are women. This is true for Long COVID as well; recent studies suggest that women who get Long COVID outnumber men who get Long COVID by as much as 4 to 1.[5]

The psychologization of women's health issues is nothing new. Filmmaker and chronic illness advocate Jennifer Brea, who was ultimately diagnosed with POTS and myalgic encephalomyelitis—once known as "chronic fatigue syndrome" and often abbreviated as ME/CFS (see page 262)—was first diagnosed with "conversion disorder," a condition in which a person has neurological symptoms that can't be explained by medical evaluation, despite her many debilitating physical symptoms. Brea's neurologist told her that her symptoms were caused by emotional trauma and that her illness had no biological cause. In her TED Talk on the subject, Brea explains that over seventy worldwide outbreaks of post-infectious diseases since 1934 have been written off as "mass hysteria," in part because they have mainly affected women.[6] "Conversion disorder," the diagnosis Brea first received, replaced the term "hysteria" in 1980. The diagnosis is still used today.

Brea's experience is backed up by study after study. In a 2015 study by the Yale School of Public Health, researchers found that gender bias often keeps women from getting proper diagnoses and treatment for coronary heart disease.[7] Sometimes this is due to women's symptoms not being "textbook" (though the textbook was literally written by men for men). Other times it's because doctors often write off women who report "anxiety" in tandem with their physical symptoms (despite the fact that anxiety is a very normal response to thinking you're having a heart attack, for example). In fact, a series of 2008 studies by psychologist Gabrielle R. Chiaramonte showed that a huge gender gap appears in correctly diagnosing and treating heart disease when women report "stress" as one of their symptoms.[8]

In a 2018 article on gender bias in medicine, journalist and author Maya Dusenbery quotes one doctor who bluntly stated: "In training, we were taught to be on the lookout for hysterical females who come to the emergency room."[9]

I'm not sharing this to discourage women, or others who face medical bias, from seeking a diagnosis; it's the opposite, in fact! It's important to understand these barriers to diagnosis so that we can advocate for ourselves in medical settings, even if that means searching multiple places before finding a health care provider who listens to and believes us. It can be demoralizing to be dismissed by health care providers, especially when we're using our already very limited energy to pursue treatment. But we are not alone, and there are medical professionals who are equipped and eager to help us. For some, there is certainly gender bias at work. For others, it is simply a matter of lack of knowledge. When I shared my dysautonomia diagnosis with my primary care physician who'd repeatedly insisted I was dealing with anxiety after COVID, she said she'd only heard of POTS once—there was a single question about it on a test she'd taken in medical school.

Because dysautonomia cannot be detected with routine testing, doctors rely on tilt table tests, which are performed at many hospitals worldwide. During a tilt table test, a patient lies on a table that raises their body from horizontal to vertical, to mimic standing straight up, and measures their heart rate and blood pressure. Patients often faint, even if they have never fainted before, because they can't call upon the physical coping mechanisms they've put into place over the years, like sitting or lying down, crossing their legs or fidgeting. Patients often report intense fatigue for a few days after the test, but an IV of saline solution can sometimes mitigate the onset of malaise. (In everyday conversation, *malaise* usually simply means a sense of discontent or the feeling of being rundown; in dysautonomia and ME/CFS communities, post-exertional malaise, or PEM, refers to the often-debilitating escalation of symptoms—or even the onset of new symptoms—that follows even the slightest bit of too much activity. PEM is also sometimes referred to as post-exertional symptom exacerbation, or PESE.)

If a patient's symptoms are in-line with standard dysautonomia symptoms, and other conditions have been ruled out, a doctor might opt for a "poor man's tilt table test" in their office. During these tests, patients go from a lying position to a sitting position and a sitting position to a standing position while wearing a simple pulse oximeter on their finger. My cardiologist was able to diagnose me based on my symptoms and several videos I'd taken of myself doing my own poor man's tilt table test at home, which we were able to easily replicate in her office.

While some health care providers are familiar with dysautonomia, it's more likely that you will need to see either a cardiologist or neurologist who specializes in dysautonomia for quicker diagnosis and more in-depth treatment. Specialists can be found by utilizing advocacy network directories or asking for suggestions in online support groups. Facebook boasts dozens of location-specific support groups hosted by Dysautonomia International, where patients share advice and medical professional recommendations.

Treating Dysautonomia

There is no known cure for dysautonomia, and symptom severity varies from person to person and often changes its manifestation over time. Because of this and the many causes of autonomic dysfunction, there's no one-size-fits-all treatment. Most health care providers try both pharmacological treatments and lifestyle-based treatments, working with patients to find a mix-and-match regimen that allows them to manage their specific symptoms best. For patients whose dysautonomia is secondary to another disease, it's imperative to treat the primary condition with a specialist to get the most out of dysautonomia treatment.

Lifestyle Treatments

Avoid triggering environments and activities: It's common for people with dysautonomia to feel much worse standing still than moving around. Washing dishes at the sink, for example, may cause more lightheadedness and a more rapid heartbeat than taking a walk. It's also common for hot environments to exacerbate symptoms. Standing in the shower is notoriously difficult, for example. The best course of action is to simply avoid these triggers, but that's not always—or even usually—possible. If you find it necessary to be in an environment that makes your dysautonomia worse, try countering the negative effects. Consider investing in a shower stool so you can actually enjoy what is usually a relaxing activity, or a bar stool to place near the counters in your kitchen so you can sit when you're prepping meals. Many people have also found it helpful to purchase a cane with a foldout seat, or portable camping stool for trips to the grocery store, doctor's office, or waiting on the sidewalk for an Uber. Always plan ahead for needing to sit down!

Compression gear: Abdominal binders and compression socks or stockings are a first-line suggestion by every health care provider who treats dysautonomia. These garments help with blood pooling, which helps keep many dysautonomia symptoms in check. As with all treatments for managing orthostatic intolerance, there's no surefire type of compression that works best. Prescription compression socks and stockings require a doctor's note and a professional fitting; while this style of compression offers fewer options, the garments are often covered by insurance, and you can be sure you're getting the right fit and strength of compression for your needs. Compression socks are also widely available from athletic and leisure-wear companies. These non-prescription options allow you to choose from a variety of colors, sizes, and materials, and often online. However, they don't offer as much compression as prescription garments. Compression calf sleeves, yoga pants, and even shorts are also options. As for which option works best—as my cardiologist says—it's whatever compression gear you'll actually wear.

Postural adaptations: Some people with dysautonomia simply cannot stand or sit up without the assistance of a mobility aid. For others, making postural adaptations can make a huge difference in the length of time you can be upright. You can try elevating the head of your mattress 10 to 15 degrees to keep your head above your heart while you sleep. Try crossing your legs while you're standing, squatting occasionally, placing one leg on a chair while you're standing, keeping your knees close to your chest in a chair while sitting, leaning down in your chair, or leaning forward while sitting or standing. These movements can help reduce blood pooling and help pump blood back up toward your head, which can help alleviate symptoms.

Hydration and salt: Electrolytes are a key component of managing dysautonomia. Increasing your fluid intake increases your blood volume, which allows more blood to circulate between your heart and your brain. Increased salt intake both increases blood pressure in patients with hypotension and encourages your body to retain the extra fluids you're adding to it. Water is great, but oral rehydration solutions are even better. Some prominent companies that market to dysautonomia patients—like Liquid I.V.—even offer significant discounts to patients with diagnoses like POTS. (While most of the suggestions on this non-pharmacological list are fine to try on your own, you should consult with your doctor before increasing your salt intake, especially if you or anyone in your family has a history of high blood pressure.)

External temperature regulation: While most dysautonomia patients have a hard time tolerating heat, many have a hard time regulating their bodies in cold weather as well. If you're leaving your house, you'll always want to dress in layers, and, if possible, with an additional resource to help counteract the outside temperature, like an ice scarf or ice vest, or microwavable/disposable hand warmers. Because people with dysautonomia often tend to experience adrenaline surges while they sleep, which leave them waking up covered in sweat, it's also important to make sure you have a variety of sleeping covers to choose from and access to both a fan and a heating pad.

Physical therapy: Exercise is a tricky pickle for people with dysautonomia. Because many people who have dysautonomia also have ME/CFS, it is imperative that patients learn to pace themselves and not get caught in the "boom or bust" cycle that occurs when post-exertional malaise (PEM) follows activity. However, patients with POTS often report a much better quality of life when they're able to do some exercise regularly. The best way to find this balance is to work with a ME/CFS or dysautonomia-literate physical therapist, or one who has been trained to work with Long COVID patients and understands PEM. More and more physical therapists are being trained to work with people who have Long COVID. When choosing a physical therapist, it's important to get references from other Long COVID patients, if possible. Above all, remember that you are the authority on your body; if a physical therapist is pushing you to do any exercises that cause PEM—or any other physical, mental, or emotional stress that worsens your condition—stop immediately. If physical therapy is not an option, finding your baseline—the amount and intensity of activity you can do without causing PEM—is your best bet. If you stick to your baseline, you may find it slowly moving in a better direction.

Heart rate and blood pressure monitoring: Heart rate and blood pressure monitoring are especially important during the early days of treating dysautonomia, as you nail down your personal baseline for activity and avoid crashing. There are seemingly infinite ways to take your vitals these days, from trendy smart watches that'll also allow you to check your email, to watches paired with a chest strap that will alert you if your heart rate goes over a certain threshold. You can also use a simple pulse oximeter that costs less than ten dollars. I did the "poor man's tilt table test" that my cardiologist used to diagnose my dysautonomia with a pulse oximeter I bought at the local drug store for five bucks. Monitoring your heart rate and blood pressure will help you tell whether or not your lifestyle adjustments and medications are working and will help you build a better picture of what your body is capable of doing and where it needs more attention.

Meditation and breathing exercises: Meditation and breathwork help our bodies remain in a more parasympathetic state (rather than the fight-or-flight state of the sympathetic nervous system). Because dysautonomia causes our bodies' adrenaline responses to go berserk, and because we're often releasing adrenaline into our bloodstream simply by standing up, it's a great idea to help train the mind and body to get back to a "rest-and-digest" state as soon as possible. Meditation is proven to help with neuroplasticity, creating new pathways between our brains' neurons to help us function in a more relaxed state. This is a nice counter to the way dysautonomia disrupts communication between our neurons, and it provides mental and emotional relaxation to a body that is constantly overstressed. Meditation cannot cure dysautonomia; like the other treatments mentioned here, it's a technique to help manage the symptoms.

Pharmacological Treatments

While no medication can cure dysautonomia, there are several types of medications that can be used to help manage symptoms.

Medications that slow down heart rate: Three of the most commonly prescribed medications for dysautonomia are propranolol, metoprolol (both beta-blockers), and ivabradine. All three slow down heart rate and lower blood pressure. Beta-blockers also interfere with the body's release and response to epinephrine and norepinephrine. If hypotension is one of your symptoms, you may need to take a second medication to counter the lowered blood pressure caused by these drugs.

Medications that constrict blood vessels: Midodrine is the most common alpha antagonist prescribed for dysautonomia. It narrows blood vessels and allows blood to get back to the heart and reach the brain. It can cause or exacerbate high blood pressure, so you should monitor yours while on this medication.

Medications that increase blood volume: Fludrocortisone helps the body retain salt, which helps keep blood volume at a more appropriate level. It's a synthetic steroid that doesn't have the same side effects as more commonly used steroids like prednisolone, which can cause fluid retention, high blood pressure, mood swings, weight gain, and gastrointestinal upset. Prednisone is another steroid that is also generally not recommended for long-term use, as it can increase the risk of infections. Desmopressin is a steroid that helps the body retain salt by slowing down urine production. Sodium and potassium levels must be monitored regularly with the use of these drugs.

Selective serotonin reuptake inhibitors (SSRIs) and serotonin-noradrenaline reuptake inhibitors (SNRIs): Because recent research suggests that serotonin is a component in the control of heart rate and blood pressure, selective serotonin reuptake inhibitors (SSRIs) and serotonin-noradrenaline reuptake inhibitors (SNRIs) are often useful in helping to manage dysautonomia. The Cleveland Clinic estimates that one third of people who are diagnosed with a life-changing chronic illness experience symptoms of depression, which often include feelings of deep sadness and despair, weight loss or gain, disturbances in sleep, feelings of worthlessness, apathy, and even thoughts of suicide. SSRIs and SNRIs have the added bonus of treating anxiety and depression, which sometimes follow a dysautonomia diagnosis.

Birth control: Most people who have dysautonomia struggle with blood volume, and if they menstruate, they feel this loss of blood during menstruation acutely. Dysautonomia symptoms are exacerbated during the menstrual cycle, and people also report a worsening of common menstruation symptoms like bloating, cramps, muscle aches, headaches, and gastrointestinal upset. Birth control—particularly continuous hormonal birth control, which does not allow the body to have a period—can help alleviate these symptoms. Oral birth control can also raise blood pressure, which is helpful for those with hypotension.

Stimulants: Because dysautonomia often causes severe fatigue, some doctors will recommend stimulants like modafinil or Adderall. While these medications can help with some of the constant tiredness and cognition issues caused by dysautonomia, they can also mask your body's need for rest, which can cause serious repercussions if you do suffer from the type of post-exertional malaise that accompanies ME/CFS. They can also exacerbate dysautonomia symptoms like racing heartbeat and tachycardia.

While many cardiologists and neurologists who treat dysautonomia are happy to work with you to manage all the prescriptions you need, you might need to seek help from other specialists if you have gastrointestinal issues or migraines. Further tests and imaging might need to be done for each of those, and health care professionals who specialize in them—especially those who are dysautonomia literate—are often able to prescribe medications to help with pain and nausea and also offer advice about diet and routine. For example, GI symptoms might need to be diagnosed and managed by a gastroenterologist or dietician. Migraines might need to be treated by a neurologist who is a headache specialist.

Living with a Disability

Learning to live with dysautonomia is about more than getting a diagnosis and finding the right combination of lifestyle and pharmacological treatments to help manage it. For most people, dysautonomia is a life-changing disorder. Once we're hit with it, it's often harder to sustain our current level of employment, due to both physical and cognitive fatigue. Relationships become more complicated, as we need more accommodations and are often unable to offer time or emotional support to our friends and family. Our lives become more expensive as we visit countless specialists and try many treatments. And as these things shift, so do our identities. In addition to struggling to stand up, we also find ourselves struggling with intense grief over what we've lost and grappling with what it means to be a person living with a disability in an ableist world.

Some dysautonomia patients will get completely better over time. Some will progress slowly to a better baseline. Some will not get better or will get progressively worse. And the spectrum of disability for patients ranges from very mild to very debilitating. Often, dysautonomia symptoms ebb and flow. Some of us can work and attend school; some of us cannot. Some of us can have active social lives; others are housebound. Some of us can exercise; some of us can't get out of bed.

Many patients even lose friends and family, who, at best, can't understand what we're going through, or, at worst, like so many health care providers, simply don't believe that our lives could be turned upside down by some kind of post-viral disorder. People living with dysautonomia often, ironically, find themselves with secondary anxiety and depression, the very thing doctors tried to diagnose us and dismiss us with in the beginning.

Taking care of our mental health becomes as important as taking care of our physical health. Finding a therapist who specializes in chronic illness and disability has been a game-changer for me. I've never even met my therapist. We communicate solely by written chat because my cognition can't stand up to an hour-long Zoom every week. But she has helped me grieve and redefine myself. She has helped me adapt my relationships by setting boundaries and advocating for my needs and has guided me in dealing with the immense guilt I feel for what I can no longer do and how it affects me and everyone around me. She has even helped me start dreaming for a different future, one I'd never planned on having but find myself excited about nonetheless. Learning to manage my physical symptoms as best as I can was only half my battle; the other half was learning how to be—and be proud—of the new me.

If therapy isn't an option for you, there are many vital support groups where Long COVID and dysautonomia patients can share their experiences, while seeking and giving support to others who are going through the same thing and working collectively as chronic illness activists to affect change. COVID has become a mass disabling event; we are not alone. There are so many people who came before us and so many who will come after us. As we look for answers and wait for more research, there is great comfort in the community we have built with one another.

The most important lessons I have learned from having Long COVID are to stand up for myself with everyone from doctors to coworkers, to keep trying new treatments until I find what works for me, and to not be afraid to lean on the advice of those who've been doing this work before COVID ever existed. As you continue on your Long COVID journey, you'll discover what your important lessons are, too.

Survival Tips

- Dysautonomia is a group of medical conditions caused by dysregulation of the autonomic nervous system, the part of your nervous system that controls the things your body does that you don't think about. That includes breathing, digestion, heart rate, blood pressure, body temperature, sleep cycles, bladder function, and hormonal function.

- The list of dysautonomia symptoms is long, varied, and often evolving.

- Cardiologists and neurologists are the types of doctors who usually diagnose dysautonomia.

- To check to see if you have Postural Orthostatic Tachycardia Syndrome (POTS), you can replicate a "poor man's tilt table test" at home by measuring your heart rate as you go from lying down to standing up. If your heart rate increases 30 beats per minute within ten minutes, you likely have POTS.

- Dysautonomia cannot be cured, but it can be managed with medications and lifestyle adjustments to help mitigate some of the symptoms.

- Common lifestyle treatments include increasing fluid and salt intake, drinking electrolytes, wearing compression socks or stockings, and avoiding triggering environments and activities.

- Dysautonomia can also be managed with medications that slow down heart rate, constrict blood vessels, and increase blood volume.

- Adjusting to life with dysautonomia can be hard, but people with disabilities can and do lead fulfilling, happy lives. Working with a therapist who specializes in chronic illness can be one of the most helpful ways to manage your new life.

CHAPTER 3

COVID Can't Be Outpaced

Learning Pacing and Radical Rest

Pato Hebert

Pacing: A self-management practice and strategy for activity. Chronically ill people who pace well are active when able, and rest when tired. We may plan extra rest ahead of and after strenuous activities.

Spoon Theory: A metaphor that uses spoons as visual tools to conceptualize units of mental or physical energy available for daily activities and tasks, developed by Christine Miserandino. Spoon theory is a helpful tool for chronically ill people to plan what they will spend our limited energy on and generally involves interspersing energy-draining activities with periods of rest.[1]

Post-Exertional Malaise (PEM): When symptoms flare up due to physical, emotional, or mental exertion; a hallmark symptom of ME/CFS; PEM is also common for COVID long-haulers, and one of the most important and difficult things for us to learn to manage and prevent.[2]

Stop: To cause to give up or change a course of action; to keep from carrying out a proposed action.[3]

Rest: Freedom from activity or labor; a state of motionlessness or inactivity; peace of mind or spirit; something used for support.[4]

Pace: Rate of movement; rate of progress; an example to be emulated; to set or regulate the pace of.[5]

Feeling Outpaced

I have been sick since March 2020. One of the most important yet difficult things for me to learn and practice has been pacing—proceeding with daily activities when I have the energy to do so, resting when the energy isn't there, and planning and adjusting my days with this rhythm in mind. This is an ongoing challenge due to my own ableist ideas about effort and worth, and because of the different paces at which my long-hauling symptoms have appeared, ebbed, reemerged, and confounded. Even writing this essay and meeting my deadlines have been challenging. COVID likes romping around and enjoying itself all over our long-hauling bodily systems. It ain't fun.

"Why are my guts clenching and on fire?" I'd already been sick for ~~sick~~ six months when this question led me back to urgent care. My first trip to urgent care was in April 2020, a month into my illness. My lungs were tight and getting tighter. Several months, chest X-rays, gentle walks and piles of inhalers later, my lungs seemed to have improved—just as my guts were getting worse.

Sick for six months, the previous paragraph says. But at first, I wrote *sick for sick months*. Then I tried to rewrite it and it came out *six for sick months*. This unwanted cognitive confusion happens all the time, still. Words slip in and out of one another, alternately entangled and playing peek-a-boo. It makes writing or public speaking or trying to share intimate thoughts with loved ones rather interesting. Often the mix-ups are incorrect homonyms. While talking, I mix up words that start with the same ~~later~~ letter or are distant relatives that share a syllable with similar vowels. Sometimes, it's just a misplaced letter or two that changes the entire word, derailing it from my intended meaning. Occasionally, there isn't even a mistaken word to be retrieved. In my head I can see a consonant or hear a sound, but there's no word there to be shared.

When I can, I keep notes of these jumbles on my phone, a poem that incrementally evolves in juxtaposed parts:

dimension dementia

whole hole

stick stink

mix mask

overdoes overdoses

art heart

sick six

later letter

I regularly find my draft emails and papers full of these slippages. I also find that I can lose all track of time. I lose track all the time. These are some of the ways I feel outpaced by the virus and its aftereffects. It always feels like COVID is ahead of me. So, I stopped thinking of being sick as something to be defeated. Or some kind of irrevocable loss. Or even as something that can be fully understood. Mostly I have endeavored to simply be with it, to make room for it. Buddhism has long guided me in such practices, ~~leaning~~ learning to give things space and pace, place and time.

Making space and practicing pacing have also meant learning the churning of my long-hauling guts. I spent months with my insides episodically pressurized and aflame, especially if I wasn't extremely careful about what I ate or drank. So, more than a year after first seeking care for the painful rumbles, I finally had surgery. It was originally scheduled for December 2020, only to be postponed at the last minute due to the winter surge of 2020. I feared it would be canceled again in the Omicron surge of 2021. But the cuts and pokes and snips occurred, and with them went my sack of sludge 'n' stones, as I'd come to call my gallbladder.

Stop. Rest. Pace.

I have had to learn that recalibration is more important than rigid notions of recuperation. I have had to recalibrate my habits and expectations, my ways of being. I have had to learn to pace. I haven't always understood the rhythms of pacing and its vital importance for long-haulers. For guidance, I turned to the wisdom of other warriors with chronic illness, and the work of #MEAction, an advocacy group and global movement for health justice.

Collective organizing first introduced me to the efforts of #MEAction. The ME in their name is not a shouting, all-caps individual self, of course, but rather the shorthand for myalgic encephalomyelitis, a complex illness that can cause extreme fatigue that does not simply improve with rest. I learned about #MEAction through the dynamic organizing that is happening between communities of ME, COVID, HIV, and disability activists. Even though ~~are~~ our more coordinated efforts are in the early years of gaining greater momentum and shared traction, we are not mutually exclusive communities. People living with chronic illnesses compare notes on gaslighting, stigma, workplace or dating challenges, strategies for advocacy, and policy changes.

I first wrote *are* in place of *our*. Ironic, given that I find meaning in my relationships with others. I have tools for grappling with long-hauling because I have been shaped by organizing, learning and playing with others. I am the political progeny of decades of HIV organizing, primarily with queer communities of color. This work has taught me about harm reduction and doula-ing, sex-positivity and strengths-based approaches to community and care. It has also blessed me by bringing countless amazing, resilient, brilliant, courageous, irreverent everyday folks, activists and organizers into my life. Some of these people are also living with ME/CFS or other chronic illnesses and disabilities. The ME/CFS community knows all about fatigue and pacing, gaslighting by health care providers and loved ones alike, and the urgent need for high-quality research, treatment, resources, and mobilization.

#MEAction's latest and ongoing campaign astutely links some of the bodily symptoms and structural conditions shared between living with ME/CFS and long-hauling with COVID. This aligned understanding of daily survival skills, community building, and advocacy strategies is invaluable—as is their call to "tell those with Long COVID to STOP. REST. PACE." Since learning of this campaign, I've been trying to enact its guiding wisdom in my daily life. This gave me the idea to structure this essay around the practices of STOP, REST, and PACE, with an eye toward naming some of what has been helpful and what has been hard.

COVID's Confusions

STOP

COVID confuses me. Even though I'd read #MEAction's reminder to STOP. REST. PACE, I had mistakenly remembered the first step as *pause*. It's almost as if I stubbornly wanted to be able to keep going after just a little break, as though I'd conflated STOP and REST into something faster, easier, a mere transition in the real action of living. But when you're long-hauling, it's not enough to pause. Pausing can help as a first step, but it's not enough. It's not a STOP. What are the harmful habits I must stop (cease)? What are the new habits I must build to learn how to STOP? How best to PACE?

As my long-hauling condition improves—unevenly, slowly, incompletely—it's tempting and exciting to want to rev up again. To exert myself in exercise, or agree to a social engagement, or say yes to a writing opportunity like this one.

Stopping, ~~reacting~~ resting and pacing can be tough for any of us who are work-aholics, perfectionists, or people pleasers. If we struggle with ego. If we don't reckon with our ableism. If we're working class, overachievers, immigrants, or survivors surviving. STOP is counter to drive. STOP can seem counter to old habits of survival. Yet often long-hauling is not about do or go. It's not even about pause. It's about STOP. I seem to have to learn this time and time again, with every crash or fogbank, every flat and blah day. I often react instead of just stopping, or better yet, resting.

REST

This reminds me of twelve-step wisdom passed on to me years ago by a friend as they worked through some of their issues. My friend taught me the acronym of HALT and its related practices. They told me that we often make unhealthy choices when we are hungry, angry, lonely, or tired (HALT). Long-hauling can leave you feeling any combination of these—and sometimes all four. It can also mess with your decision making. I try to remember the STOP in #MEAction's practice, and in that stopping, consider the HALT. Have I eaten anything nour-ishing? Am I angry? Lonely? Tired?

Of these, tired is my most common. I'm privileged to have enough food to eat, even if I am sometimes too tired to make it or take care with it. I have a wide and deep support network, even though I'm often too wiped out to activate it or too overwhelmed by social interaction and expectations. I'm not particularly lonely, as I am an introvert who loves solitude and who is blessed to have many different kinds of multidirectional love and care in my life.

In a given moment I can certainly be hungry, angry, or lonely, and I can act in ways that are not caring for my being and those around me. But my biggest challenge with long-hauling is fatigue. Early on, it was straight-up exhaustion. It could flatten me in an instant, seemingly out of nowhere. Even getting to the bed was sometimes impossible. I still experience one or two days a week where I am very, very tired. More often, there is just mental flatness, a ~~loek~~ lack of vi-tality and drive, difficulty sleeping, constant ambient fatigue.

This perceived lack can stop me in my tracks, but I try to reconceptualize it as something more than a lack. "You're not at full capacity," a friend says over brunch. I counter that this now *is* my full capacity. This long-hauling body is full of new limits and difficult lessons. Rest doesn't often turbocharge me, or even readily replenish me. But rest can bring me back into the present and create a bit of spaciousness that helps me be, especially when I have no motivation to go or do. This difference between being and doing is something I've learned in Buddhism. Practicing ways of being without doing, ways of being without trying (exerting, asserting, controlling), ways of being without expectation, is much easier said than done. Buddhist teachings about resting and refuge invert the Western and capitalist productivity demand of "Don't just sit there, do something!" Meditation offers something very different: "Don't just do something; sit there." Sit here. With all this. Slow down. Rest.

As long-haulers, it's important for us to learn to recognize our triggers and develop new rhythms. When I get spaced out, lost in a fog, sometimes I try to pace out. By this I mean I try to come back to breathing, limit inputs (phone, tasks, frets), simplify sensations. If I can, I sit or lie down. If I can, I close my eyes. If I can, I slow down. Maybe this is a form of resting, though if I'm spinning it can feel much more like a somewhat desperate rescue mission.

PACE

My HIV-work-husband George Ayala and I have been collaborating for over twenty years. We've developed local programs and services with queer communities of color, spearheaded cutting-edge research, created campaigns, made art and publications, and played a part in building global movements for health and human rights. Years into this collective effort, he learned that he has multiple sclerosis (MS). He calls MS his uninvited guest, sends me playlists from his infusion sessions, selfies with IV drips and slightly sarcastic smiles.

Early in my days with COVID, George counseled me about pacing, preparation, and crashes. He shared that when he has a big presentation or stressful meeting ahead, he tries to clear out some space on the calendar before and after whatever he knows will take a lot of out him. We still talk about these long on-ramps and off-ramps, the ways that chronic illness and middle age no longer allow for rapid lane changes and trying to cover large distances in short amounts of time. Pacing ain't always pretty. It's often frustrating and confusing, especially at first.

George reminds me that slowing down is also part of the aging process. One of its gifts is that we can notice new things and experience the world differently. I have often felt that COVID took years off my life. Not just the lost time with loved ones and important family trips that fell away during sheltering in place, but whole years off of the back end of my life. I can't actually know that my life will now be cut short due to COVID, and I certainly hope it's not true. But this, too, has impacted my sense of pacing. I don't want to be in frantic or scarcity modes of living. And I don't have the stamina or energy to try to cram things in. So, I notice and experience what I can. Sometimes pacing is about quality not quantity. I am slowly learning new qualities of care.

Syncopated Pacing

STOP

My first thoughts upon receiving Fiona Lowenstein's invitation to write this chapter were that I didn't have time and energy, and was not the right person. I feel like a bumbling novice around pacing. But I realized that being honest about this can be part of my contribution. Pacing is a learning process. It takes practice, mistakes, support. So, I heeded Fiona's suggestion to consider engaging with the wisdom of #MEAction.

While writing this essay, I've simultaneously been working on a large solo art exhibition about long-hauling. *Lingering* is the title. It's a nod to COVID's ongoing presence and impact in our lives, and the reckoning that comes with dismantling one's own ableism when you begin to experience and comprehend chronic illness.

REST

COVID's pace can feel relentless. It's so good at both syncopating and overwhelming. It can come at you nonstop but also sneak up on you in new rhythms and worries, intense or strange symptoms. For me these include frequent bouts of crying due to pseudobulbar affect (a neurological condition of sudden or uncontrollable laughing or crying), phantom smells of burning wood and wires, common and difficult sleep disruptions, dropping and breaking dishes while scrubbing in the sink, or clumsily tipping a plate, and with it half of dinner. It feels like COVID fucks with everything. Sometimes it makes pacing in day-to-day rhythms seem impossible. Flare-ups, crashes, fractured sleep, fog—they've all continued to pester me.

I've tried many tricks with these symptoms—I stopped returning their texts, unfollowed them on social media, tried having heart-to-hearts, tried calling them in, then out, tried ignoring them, and tried holding boundaries. But these bullies are very codependent, and sometimes even cruel. How does one rest when rest itself does not want you? I've been thinking of asking my neurologist this.

PACE

At least last week's quarterly appointment, my neurologist agreed with me that I should try going back on a med that helps with headaches and, anecdotally, seems to aid some long-haulers with our sleep. I didn't find it all that effective after a few months of taking it in 2021. But now, after weeks of shallow "sleeps" ranging from three and a half to six hours, I'm once again willing to try it. At the appointment she runs me through a battery of physical exams. We've been doing these for a year and a half now. The first time was by video. But this time, we are in a small examination room. She has me walk across the room on my tiptoes, then return on my heels, then walk the linoleum floor in a straight line, putting one foot in front of the other, like in a field sobriety test.

After I waddle my way across the room, she asks with a hint of encouragement in her voice, "Remember what it was like when I asked you to do these before?" I don't. I have a vague recollection of it being sobering. But I can't remember much beyond that, or whether it was in 2020 or 2021, or if it included other physical tests. These gaps in time are part of why it's helpful to my pacing to check in with myself, loved ones, and professionals at least every three months to see how I'm doing. The neurologist says I am making progress. I want to trust this.

In the space of a given day, or even week or month, I can't really gauge things. But when I pause or check in and compare things to how they were three months prior, I can better feel and see the shifts. Six-month or one-year reviews offer even greater perspective. I need the scale of these larger intervals to more accurately assess. If you find yourself getting lost or overwhelmed in the granular, you might consider keeping a tracker for symptoms and energy levels. This can help you and your support ~~symptoms~~ systems take stock and make adjustments over time.

Conundrums of Care

STOP

This semester, for the first time, I am teaching a class on comics, disability, and illness. During last week's class, students wrestled with the complexities of care, accountability, and support. They were asking questions laden with both expectations and compassion. "What do we owe someone who is in need?" "What do we owe ourselves when we are at our limits?" One student brought up the analogy of the emergency instructions that we hear just prior to a flight taking off. She said she never used to understand the guidance to place your own oxygen mask first before trying to help a child or someone else. When she was younger, she thought this guidance was selfish and strange. But as she got older, she came to realize that if you don't secure your own oxygen, you may become incapacitated before you can help anyone else or yourself. You have to stop and tend to your own mask first.

REST

I chose to go public right after I tested positive. Many people said I was the first infected person they knew, and in addition to lots of texts, calls, and care packages wishing me well and sending me support, I also had people eager for nitty-gritty details. Very little was known about the disease, and they wanted the body's frontline dispatches. At first, I tried to do my best to describe what I was going through, to find words for the symptoms and reassurance for their concerns. At the end of one day, I was incredibly exhausted in ways I did not yet understand. I wondered to myself, *All I've done was talk. Why am I so wiped out?* I returned one last friend's call, someone who'd nearly pleaded for me to do so, "just so I can hear your voice and know that you're okay." I tried, and quickly hit the wall even harder. I did my best to be polite and reassuring, to respond to a few questions and also still signal that I was wiped out. "Could you just stay on a little longer and describe a bit more about what you're feeling?" they asked. But this body was not a news feed or a research finding. "I'm really sorry," I mumbled, "but I really can't. I have to rest."

Those were the days when I would completely shut down mid-sentence. I had never experienced the intensity of all-consuming fatigue. I used to have deep reservoirs of energy, many extra gears. COVID crushed my ableism and false sense of agency alike. Now when the crashes come, yielding is the only thing possible.

PACE

I don't quite know how to hold boundaries around people wanting things. But my fellow long-haulers teach me. Last night I presented on a webinar with long-hauler and longtime community health organizer Lisa Hayeem Carver. She shared that quiet is one of her tips for navigating long-hauling. She said she can't engage people like she used to—it's too tiring and overwhelming. She told us that many of her friendships have devolved because people didn't understand her need for space and quiet, and took it personally when she could no longer socialize or meet up like they used to, prior to COVID. Her voice was both sad and matter-of-fact as she said this, but it became spacious when she told us how important quiet has become to her well-being. Her wisdom cautions us against the trap of isolation yet toward the restorative practice of quiet. I so appreciated being in her company, absorbing her testimony and wisdom. We long-haulers need one another.

I remembered a long call last Thanksgiving, which I spent away from blood family. I was already tired that night when my siblings lovingly FaceTimed me. I was okay for the first thirty or forty minutes, enjoying being silly, catching up, seeing faces and the march of time pixelated in my hand. My parents got patched in. I hadn't seen them in over five months and wouldn't for another seven. My tía joined from Virginia. I hadn't spent time with her in four years. I was supposed to take my mom to visit her in May of 2020 so that they could have some sister time. COVID obliterated that carefully coordinated reunion, and that made this holiday FaceTime feel more precious and pressurized. I hung in there as best I could, but having multiple animated voices ~~taking~~ talking simultaneously ended up fraying my nerves. I started becoming overwhelmed, increasingly shutdown and withdrawn from the conversation. I felt too self-conscious to say I needed to get off, though nobody would have cast aspersions. Still, I didn't want to disrupt the party, and I didn't really understand what was happening until it was too late.

My ability to show up and hold space for folks I care about has been profoundly challenged—whether it's something as simple as a holiday call or as confounding as taking a loved one to the emergency room while being sick myself. I try to trust that if I am long-hauling it also means that I am still alive, and that meaningful relationships can endure for just as long as COVID does. But I can no longer contribute to these relationships in the ways that I used to. This excavates my ego and harasses my heart in ways that are painful and stark.

I call this the conundrum of care, the reality that you cannot always be there. There have been moments where I've shown up in support and then later paid the price with nasty crashes and relapses. One of the hardest parts of long-hauling amid the pandemic is that even if most people are not long-haulers, everyone has been impacted by this horrific pandemic. So, the existing circuitries and rhythms of reciprocity and care can become fried. Everybody needs more support, more understanding, more resources and love. We are burned out.

Walk Out of Here

STOP

The doctor told me that after surgery it would help to walk as much as I can. "You're going to walk out of the hospital, so you can take a walk later that same day of surgery if you want." Technically, I am wheeled out. But a few hours later, here I am at the park, on my feet, wobbly, shaking, constipated from the pain meds, but moving—slowly and safely. My entire abdominal wall hurts with each step. It takes all of my focus to move. I am groggy but determined to navigate the uneven terrain, to breathe through repeated pain. I need the land and breeze, the birds and the other beings—some older and stronger, some younger and more vulnerable than me. I need reminders of different priorities, different scales of time.

REST

Three days later I am able to shower. I've been resting and walking and watching TV. After the gift of warm water on my skin, I pause before exiting, remember to move mindfully and steady myself on the shower frame, gently raise my legs one at a time to clear the glass door and tub's edge, and probe cautiously for the cushioned mat on the cold floor outside and below.

More days pass and eventually the bandages can be peeled off. I rub some ointment and cocoa butter on my scar tissue. There are four thick memories raised upon my torso that mark the probe's retreat, the surgeon's stitches, the flesh's capacity to mend—the healing power of rest.

PACE

I'm folding laundry now. It sat untouched in the basket for days. Actually, first it sat in the dryer (something I'm privileged to have in my apartment), then it was in the basket, now, finally, I am folding. For some reason, I saved the yellow safety socks they'd given me at the hospital, the ones with white sticky bumps to keep me from slipping on the sterilized floor. Tears well up as I'm rolling these memories for storage. I align the two pieces, fold them into one another and torque, the ribbed texture coiling in my hand, turning on the faucet of tears a bit more with each twist.

Two Ambulance Town/Ánimo

STOP

"I feel like a sick person," one of my students says to me during office hours. "You are," I say simply, directly, lovingly, with encouragement and solidarity. "We are."

From our very first advisement session last September, we have talked together about being long-haulers. It's the new year, and we are still talking about silence and isolation, not wanting to worry or burden loved ones, the impossibility and harm of trying to carry it alone, the power of sharing.

This student's city of fifty-six thousand people in the Global South only has two ambulances. So when their lungs started shutting down and they called for emergency transport to the hospital, it took three hours for the ambulance to arrive at their home. "I thought I was going to die," they say matter-of-factly but in a near whisper. "I still haven't told my family."

This is part of why I write publicly about my messy process with COVID. This is why I started sharing via social media the day after I tested positive and why I haven't ceased. Why the collection you are holding, and in which we are meeting, matters. Individually we must always stop and take our breaks. But collectively we cannot ever stop organizing spaces and paces of care with and for one another. Each of us individually lives in unique and evolving circumstances, and we should always have the right to our respective privacy, process, and dignity. But we should never feel like we have to live in isolation to sustain these.

REST

I message my prima in Panamá to say I hope to finally visit later this year. The last time was 2007 when my abuelita was laid to rest. It's been such a long time. We were set for a historic family gathering back in June of 2020 before the pandemic made that impossible. I still don't know if a visit can occur in the coming months, but I am cautiously hopeful. She tells me how emotional it makes her to imagine finally reconnecting. My cousin knows I'm a long-hauler, and has messaged me encouragement and cariño many times. She tells me that she and her youngest both caught Omicron. I sense from between the lines of the brief note that they're okay-ish, then I get lost in a week of deadlines and tasks. I feel bad for not responding right away. This is the kind of connective tissue that long-hauling has eaten away from me. I struggle to maintain these vital capillaries of care. I finally message her back, asking how her camino de COVID is going. This time she responds with a voice memo. Just hearing her voice unleashes a tropical rainstorm of tears in me. She's fine, gratefully vaccinated and hardly impacted. Her youngest has had more bumps but is also, mostly, okay. This news is a huge relief, but it's her voice that brings out my tears. I have missed this Panamanian pacing, these sounds and inflections. It's not a long recording, but its arrival over social media means everything to me.

I feel both grateful and fatigued around the flotsam of communication that swirls in these pandemic times. Sometimes the texts and calls make it hard for me to navigate the cluttered waters, yet other times they are desperately needed lifelines that keep me tenuously and meaningfully afloat. Some hours after my gallbladder surgery, a dear, old compa, already living with HIV, texted to say that they now had COVID, too. Even talking to me overwhelmed them. I know this conundrum in my marrow. I encouraged them to rest, rest, rest, more than they think they needed, more than their habits know, more than their body allows. Rest is absolutely crucial in our first few weeks after infection.

It was raining, a rare and much needed occurrence in LA. But it also made it that much harder for them to problem-solve the compounding cascade of onset symptoms, the throbbing headaches, the need for food. I wanted badly to get them some groceries, to prep and deliver some meals. But I was only infrequently out of bed myself, mostly just for bathroom breaks and my brief daily walk post-surgery. This was my own recovery rhythm, the boundary of the body's capacity to give. I didn't say any of this. My friend didn't even know about my surgery, and there was really no point in telling them at that moment. So, I brainstormed out loud about other folks in their network who might be able to mobilize and triage on their behalf. "Honestly Pato, I'm too tired to even think about any of that right now. I'm just exhausted."

PACE

Change is sometimes small for me—very small. And that's okay. It's so important to challenge and be non-attached to hero narratives. It is also vital to be connected with others. Ableism tends to think of exertion as valiant, necessary, expected. But exertion can also do harm. This doesn't mean people are meek, that we are without ideas, strategy, conviction, effort, intention, coordination. We dose our doses of self-medication and care. Through mutual aid we help each other to pace and survive. This is vital. My friend, the harm reductionist and Bronx-based organizer Tamara Oyola-Santiago, reminds me that ~~overdoes~~ overdoses have increased intensely during the pandemic. This is a racial justice issue. The Latinx drug overdose death rate jumped 40 percent in 2020. Black people had the largest increase in overdose mortality rates in 2020, and Indigenous people experienced the highest overdose mortality rates of all. The scale of our collective suffering is immense. We must address the structural causes of this crisis as we learn how to resource and pace our response to our predicaments and pain.

Dr. Nadine Burke Harris, California's first surgeon general, announced in February 2022 that she is stepping down after three years of leading in the pandemic. She spoke of wanting to take care of herself and her family. An expert on childhood trauma and an innovator at dismantling systems of oppression and building resources for resilience with communities of color, Burke Harris warns us that COVID is "probably the greatest collective trauma of our generation." She signals that "the health consequences of this pandemic will continue long after the virus itself is contained."[6] This, too, is part of our long-hauling. Structural change, resource reallocation, and mental health support must all be significant parts of our shared pacing.

How Do(n't) You Do It?

STOP

A student has stopped by my office for the first time. We're late getting started because the previous student was late, and I'm juggling to try to see them both in rapid succession. The second student starts by asking, "How do you do it? You have Long COVID, and you understand spoons, and you're teaching and making your art and running our department. I just wanna know how you do it?" I tell her that I don't, at least not very well. My apartment is a disaster. My finances are in disarray. I'm behind on my upcoming exhibitions. I struggle with the velocity and density of life on almost any given day. This body is wracked and wrecked. I also share some of the things that appear throughout this essay, different techniques I am developing to cope and continue on. We are as adaptable and resilient as we are imperfect, I suggest, then ask how she does it—moving to a new city and starting a new grad program while living with ME/CFS. I am inspired by her work. Our exchange is rich if a little rushed, a great seed for a new working relationship. As she exits my office, she respectfully thanks me for my time (even though I was just doing my job) and says she's looking forward to class. I turn to the inbox to keep it from exploding, get lost in countless contingencies and details.

REST

Eventually, I step next door to talk to our administrative director about a few things bearing down on our week. "Do you have a minute?" I knock and ask. "Yes," she says, "but weren't you supposed to be in class 20 minutes ago?" It's early in the semester so I haven't yet normalized an internal clock for time, space, class, and pace. I'm mortified—no time to converse or rest. I'm super late for class. I'm never late for class. On time is early, I was taught. But in a hurried frenzy I make my way up the block and down to the basement where I should've been at noon. My light-skinned self is beet red and beat. But something special has happened. As I slip into the room, the preassigned student discussion leaders are already deep in dialogue. They went ahead and initiated things on their own without me. I am so grateful, relieved, impressed, proud. Our pedagogy is working. They are working, even when I am not. I almost start weeping in front of everyone.

I slink over to my customary corner of the room, bide my time for a break in the conversation to address my tardiness and make amends. Eventually I apologize profusely and explain that I didn't properly manage the cascade of backed-up appointments all morning, got confused about our start time. I'd already told them about my long-hauling at the beginning of the school year and signaled that they might encounter any number of my symptoms, from mixed-up words to low energy to fraying under too much stimulus. They are gracious and understanding. I'm too embarrassed and honest to be performing. I don't think they are either.

PACE

Some weeks later, the student describes for the class her idea for a new project, in which she would invite other people living with ME/CFS and chronic illness to share their stories in a compilation. Part of each student's proposal process is to discuss challenges or sticking points, things that they might want the group's guidance or feedback on. She reveals that she's worried about even asking other folks living with ME/CFS to participate, knowing the paradox of inviting more work from people living with chronic illness, the potential dilemma of asking them to expend their spoons. Her peers listen and encourage her to consider asking far enough in advance and inviting enough people that she'll account for the many people that may need to say no. I praise her thoughtfulness and care, and I share that what may well be a paradox and dilemma might also be an opportunity to model and enact accessible community building. I say, "If it's truly an invitation, let it be so and offer them an out. State that it's okay to say no and they should feel no pressure to participate." Together we ponder what care can look like, and the messiness of enacting it together, especially with people we might not know or know well.

A few classes later, the semester is intensifying toward its end. I'm trying to maintain enthusiasm in the room, convey lots of moving pieces and frame final papers while answering questions and holding space for everyone's anxieties. On the right side of the room a pair of students keeps talking, loudly. I try a few times to focus us, asking for one voice at a time, signaling I'll aim to get to everyone's questions as they arise. Still, the chatter persists. It's rude, but it's also just excitement and camaraderie and a need to connect. It overwhelms me as simultaneous sound streams so often and easily do now. My brain starts to melt mid-sentence and I can't function. I exhale and sternly say, "Please. If you need to work something out, please leave the room to do so. I get really easily overwhelmed with too many inputs and your conversation is making it hard for me to do my job!"

Part of pacing is knowing what you need. Another part is being honest about, asking for, and sometimes demanding what you need. Still another part is being in respectful dialogue with others, doing the slow and steady work over time to build the understanding and trust it takes to cultivate disability justice. We have to establish a sense of shared needs, mobilize and adjust resources as necessary, be accountable for missteps, allow for ouch/oops (as good facilitators and community organizers know), ask for help, genuinely give when possible, be honest when not—and learn and evolve, together. What is the pace of long-hauling possibility? What are its problems and perils? I spend the rest of the week mulling over my actions. I'm frustrated—not ashamed—at becoming overwhelmed by too much noise. I worry that my tone was too sharp and that my direction could've been more patient and still just as effective. The virus is evolving. I must, too.

Mouth Yoga

STOP

In the snarl of writing this essay, the great Buddhist monk Thich Nhat Hanh stopped breathing and began what is described as "continuation." He was ninety-five years old. Thay (or "teacher" as Hanh was lovingly called by students)—a political exile and innovator, and a man of color—guided us into working through difference while embracing interbeing without merely grasping or clinging. Across multiple continents, he shared the depths of his knowledge and gifted us practices in Vietnamese, English, and French rhythms. His teachings began to transform my life decades ago. Later, his lessons on mindfulness and breathing proved invaluable as COVID made my lungs tighter and tighter, when every breath felt far from peace. Hanh established monasteries and study centers and created spaces and communities for retreat, refuge, and replenishment. He taught of continuation, not death. It makes me reconsider STOP as continuation, not cessation.

REST

I once heard a dharma talk where Hanh reminded us: No mud, no lotus. Our growth sometimes happens in difficult circumstances. In another talk, he shared that smiling is like yoga for the mouth, food for the mood, a gift to self and others. Of course, this made me smile. From where do your smiles arise? What is the mud in which you must grow? What do you find in your COVID and pandemic breaths? What do you release?

It felt like a significant moment in my long-hauling healing when I was able to come off both the daily and the emergency asthma inhalers. During my hardest COVID days, inhaling was often much more difficult. My chest X-rays came back clear, thankfully showing no structural damage. But I could still feel the capacity of my lungs inhibited well before my body could take in enough oxygen. This gave rise to my tendency to push and exert in an effort to take in more, enough. More. Enough. So much to hold there. Anxiety also wanted in on the action.

Nearly two years later, I still have fleeting asthmatic episodes a few times a month—typically when I'm tired, self-conscious, stressed, or sometimes while

I'm climbing stairs or racing down the sidewalk. But if, in these moments, I can slow down my breathing and focus, I can find my way back to rest upon full exhale. This rest is not pressured but rather is slowed and slowly more trusting. Then I can practice pausing—resting—at the end of the exhale, extending the breath further and emptying the lungs as fully as possible without panicking that the pause will become a problem. This process then leads to a pace of breathing that is much deeper and more restorative, if still susceptible to COVID's occasional crushes.

PACE

Twice in the 2000s I was able to participate in peace walks led by Hanh and fellow monks around the perimeter of MacArthur Park, in one of the densest parts of Los Angeles. Peace walks. Walking *in* peace, not simply for peace. Something rather different from a march. We did not move along a single straight vector, but more like a circle cum weave. We moved in silence. Even the city's midday sounds seemed to quiet, though perhaps that was just our focused attention. Hanh moved very slowly, deliberately, with great intention. Peace in every step he taught, walked, embodied, invited.

When you change your usual harried gait, you inhabit your body and world differently. When you follow and deepen your breath, you inhabit the body and world differently. How do you walk in peace when COVID arrives? How do you live in peace when the bombs rain down and the troops invade? As I write, some global jurisdictions debate Omicron lockdown, and Ukraine is under violent siege. In his 2002 book, *No Death, No Fear*, Hanh wrote, "This body is not me; I am not caught in this body, I am life without boundaries, I have never been born and I have never died." I have been learning how to hold (and release) this in relationship to long-hauling. I don't yet know how best to hold this in relationship to war. But many decades into study, I am still learning from Hanh's pace as a refugee of war, a lifelong activist in and for peace, a lotus in a sea of fire.

Flutterances

STOP

My exhibition installed, this essay late and not yet finished, I head up the California Central Coast on a desperately needed break with my boo. For over two decades I've come here to celebrate my birthday when time and coin allow. This is my first visit in three years. I make the pilgrimage to a grove of eucalyptus trees. This is Chumash land, and the trees are tall but do not have old history here. Colonialism brought them. But monarch butterflies have adopted and adapted to them. The grove offers shelter from wind and ample branches for clustering and care. It is an overwintering site for the monarchs as they journey on their annual migration north. When I first came in 1999, there were tens of thousands. High up in the branches they'd cluster so thick that they appeared like dense clumps of leaves. But on days when the sky is blue and the sun is bright, they delight in the warmth and take magnificent flight in all directions. It is breathtaking, breath giving.

On my nearly annual visits, I have been crestfallen to see the monarchs' numbers dwindle and then radically plummet. According to Cal Poly San Luis Obispo Professor Dennis Frey, the count was 115,000 in the winter of 1998 to 1999, when those butterflies first enthralled me. During my last visit in 2019, the count was a horrifying 3,077. But this year, for reasons scientists don't yet fully understand, there was a rebound. The monarchs' abundance is nowhere near historic levels, but it is an exciting and encouraging 22,000. They've stopped here to recharge and wait for spring. I am fortunate to join them.

REST

My neck is craned upward in wonder when I see them drop. I sense a commotion a few feet away. On the ground are two intertwined monarchs. They're not resting. At least one of them isn't. They're steadily going at it in reproductive ardor, or perhaps just sex-positive glee. There are only brief breaks as they make the dirt their den of delight. I take a video, my hands aging and unsteady, two minutes and thirty-seven shaky seconds of butterfly porn, or my own giddy gawking. They are so beautiful, the beats of their wings planar convergences of grace and power. Eventually they finish, disentangle, and rapidly ascend to the sky. I do not want to contain my smile. This gift of their company is the best birthday present, as they generously allow me to briefly visit with them in this camp along their own glorious long haul.

PACE

Not quite twenty miles north of the monarchs' encampment is an old grove of gorgeous California coastal oaks. It's usually much less crowded than the enthusiastic bustle we humans cause at the monarchs' migratory hub. The oak grove is dense and quiet, full of lichen and filtered light, thick trunks and twisting limbs. These oaks don't allow no body shaming. And if you move carefully and with respect, they might just reward you with the most spectacular sculptural experience ever. Each step shifts space and a sense of dimension. Gravity's normal rules are no longer a given amid such deep rootedness and mass, amazing arcs and undulation. Many of these magnificent beings expand as fully outward and downward as they do to the heavens. A trailer park runs along the north side of the grove, and there are large private lots to the west. On the eastern edge our belching cars disrupt in percussive whooshes and moans. But inside, the grove holds so much time, and the deeper you move toward the middle, the more still everything seems to be. The breeze is modest here, only occasionally deciding to dance with the moss. Shade predominates. I can't help but slow down.

Hay Tiempo

STOP

Back in the city, I spend some time with a former student, now a friend. They have an exciting new job that last week had them running an art fair in LA. They invite me to come visit the Hollywood hotel where the fair is staged. We haven't seen each other since before the pandemic. I notice a new tattoo on their wrist. It looks like handwriting, but I can't quite tell. It's dark where we're sitting poolside and my middle-aged eyes aren't so great. My compa tells me a story about visiting the studio of the legendary Mexican photographer Manuel Alvarez Bravo and seeing "hay tiempo" written twice just outside of his darkroom, his place of creative alchemy. "Hay tiempo"—there's time. This small and beautiful script appears across their skin in Alvarez Bravo's handwriting, a delicate single line they had inked as a reminder for the frenetic pace of the day-to-day.

REST

As we tend to one another in our spaces of mutual aid, recalibration, and care, what might we dream together? What must we make time for? What might appear here in time?

PACE

I want to give thanks for Audre Lorde, who taught us that poetry is not a luxury. I want to suggest here that pacing is not simply a luxury. That it is the vital matter of tending, contending and survival. We are so terrorized by precarity, the ways it makes time seem like a taunting scarcity. The settlers' and soldiers' advance. The border crossing or seascape imperiled yet also opened up by the night. The hounds at your heels on the underground railroad. Hunger. The frantic flight from a violent home. Stalking. Sometimes it feels like there is no breath or time. Sometimes it seems all we do is time. Our sisters and brothers and nonbinary beloveds in prison know the doing and being of time all too well, especially those who were infected in inhumane conditions and are still long-hauling on the inside.

Long COVID, chronic illness, disability, and the uneven evolution of justice can easily make the world feel stuck. All mud, no lotus? But we've been practicing elaborate pacing for centuries. Smallpox, measles, tuberculosis, HIV, and COVID have all threatened to obliterate us. Colonialism and racial capitalism conspire. Yet we remain, even thrive. Stopping, resting, and pacing can restore a sense of trust, bring clarity and energy to our organizing, reconnect us with ourselves and one another, the land, water, and sky. For this there is and must always be time.

Survival Tips

STOP

Prioritize. What's most important this week? Today? Right now?

Stop trying to be everything to everybody. You don't need to be the same kind of person, friend, or family member you were before you got COVID. Do care for others and show up when you can. But don't try to do too much, and don't be unkind to yourself or feel guilty when you have to maintain boundaries or when you have nothing to give. Minimize your exposure to social pressure and expectations. Maximize the time it takes to recognize and fulfill whatever it is you need. Multitasking is not healthy and is not your friend. Rushing creates risks. Stopping puts some space back into your long haul.

REST

Regular rest refocuses us on our needs, not our accomplishments.

Rest isn't just a break from doing. Rest is a way of being.

Rest doesn't always replenish us. But it's still necessary. We don't rest to be able to go out and do more. We rest to give our long-hauling bodies, minds, and spirits the space they need to be. Resting can reassure us that it's okay to feel run-down. Rest makes room for feeling unmotivated, unfocused or in a fog.

PACE

Pacing is care. We have to recalibrate. We have to cultivate different paces of care.

Long-hauling time is fluid, and changes depending on our needs, our spoons, our priorities and what is happening around us. You may need an entire weekend of quiet, a whole day to just do laundry, a week or month off social media, an extra-long soak in the tub, more time to prepare meals, or more honesty that you need help from your support network with the basics of daily living. You may need several months to see even minor changes, growth, or improvement. These are all healthy paces of care. Keep developing and trusting yours; keep sharing and honing them with others.

CHAPTER 4

With Disability, Comes Rights

Navigating the Financial Impacts of Long COVID

*Letícia Soares, Karyn Bishof,
and Alison Sbrana*

I f you're living with or caring for someone with Long COVID, you'll most likely find yourself struggling to make ends meet. It's incredibly challenging to be chronically ill, disabled, and financially insecure in a society that offers scarce and inadequate support to disabled people and ties personal worth to wealth and productivity. If you find yourself facing financial insecurity upon becoming chronically ill, please know first and foremost that this is due to a systemic failure and is not your individual failure. If you find yourself wondering how you got here, please know that you're not alone. This failure, unlike SARS-CoV-2, is not novel, nor does it affect a small number of people. Disabled and chronically ill people are rarely afforded the necessary protections to live, thrive, and survive, and people with invisible disabilities often face even greater stigmas and barriers to accessing the few benefits that are available.

We are three chronically ill women—Letícia Soares, Karyn Bishof, and Alison Sbrana—whose lives went from ordinary to anything but, after viral infections. Letícia and Karyn are COVID-19 long-haulers who, despite coming from very different backgrounds, found themselves struggling financially after becoming chronically ill. Here, they'll share their experiences on the financial impact of Long COVID in their lives and discuss the lack of available resources for the millions now facing disability from Long COVID. Alison lives with pre-pandemic viral-triggered ME/CFS; she'll discuss navigating disability benefits with practical resources to help you or the long-hauler in your life through this difficult, confusing, and stressful time. Like many people living with Long COVID, and the broader chronic illness and disability community, we have been left without proper social support, resources, and medical care because of inaccessible support programs and numerous barriers to care.

The financial impact of Long COVID is not negligible. For long-haulers, financial insecurity and instability happen both due to loss of income from inability to work and increased expenses associated with living with a complex and disabling chronic illness. This was the case for many chronically ill and disabled people prior to the pandemic, and people with Long COVID now face this same combination of challenges, with the additional burden of financial instability from the pandemic. Working full-time is difficult for many long-haulers, because the type and severity of Long COVID symptoms can fluctuate over time.[1] The unpredictability that comes with a relapsing-remitting illness makes it hard for long-haulers to plan their activities, even if they're just a few hours into the future. It can also be difficult for long-haulers to predict how much they'll be able to do and for how long, because many experience a worsening of symptoms after mental or physical exertion. While Long COVID can cause a great deal of physical and emotional suffering to patients, long-haulers are often misjudged as healthy, nondisabled people through outsider eyes. People living with invisible illnesses like Long COVID often face extra scrutiny when expressing their needs and health concerns. Thus, some long-haulers struggle to work at all, since it can be very difficult to find employers willing to accommodate them.

Because some illnesses and disabilities are neither obvious nor visible to outsiders, people living with invisible disabilities often struggle to be believed by friends and family, medical providers, and caseworkers who may determine disability benefits—an experience many COVID-19 long-haulers can relate to. But long-haulers aren't the first people to deal with this issue. People with ME/CFS and associated conditions share similar experiences and symptoms to some Long COVID patients and have, for years, also been left to fend for themselves both financially and medically. People with ME/CFS have also experienced disbelief from the medical establishment.

ME/CFS is a serious neuroimmune disease that affects some COVID-19 long-haulers. The defining feature of ME/CFS is the worsening of symptoms after physical, mental, or emotional activity, a phenomenon known as post-exertional malaise (PEM). ME/CFS also includes symptoms like brain fog, muscle and joint pain, headaches, unrefreshing sleep, and dizziness or symptom worsening when standing or sitting up (orthostatic intolerance).[2] Prior to the COVID-19 pandemic, about two and a half million Americans were living with ME/CFS, making it more than twice as prevalent as multiple sclerosis.[3] People with ME/CFS have been met with financial loss, stigma, and social systems unprepared to meet their needs. But we're here to tell you that you can find guidance and support in our community of disabled and chronically ill people—support that can help you survive financially while learning to live with a chronic, disabling illness.

While our lives, health issues, and finances differ, all three of us live the daily reality of chronic illness and financial struggle. We know that, in many cases, Long COVID patients are new to chronic illness and disability. Navigating these resources for the first time can be overwhelming—especially when you're dealing with fatigue, brain fog, and PEM. When you have to pace to manage your PEM, your energy is your most valuable currency. We live in bodies that run low in supply no matter the demand, so we know that navigating disability and social support systems can be energy-draining, and even prohibitive for some. We also know that systemic racism, sexism, and ableism can cause and exacerbate traumas associated with becoming newly sick or disabled and trying to access support. The stories, knowledge, and support of disability activists who came before us have been some of the most powerful sources of resilience and survival within our community. Thus, we share our own stories in the hope we can do the same for others. Our insights are based on our lived experiences in the United States and Canada, but we hope that patients everywhere will find something relatable and helpful here.

On the Burden of Proof and Finding Resilience in Community

Letícia Soares

It was 3 AM when SARS-CoV-2 made its unsettling debut—a migraine. *So weird,* I thought. I couldn't help but immediately fear COVID-19, and rightfully so. It was April 2020: Baking yeast was a commodity and masking wouldn't even be mandatory for another six months in Ontario, Canada. Because my job in academia as a postdoctoral researcher allowed me some flexibility, I had the privilege of opting into self-isolation before the province declared a state of emergency. When that migraine first appeared in the middle of the night, I had been self-isolating for three weeks.

I remember those three weeks so vividly. My days were filled with anxiety, keeping track of infection and hospitalization rates. I spent hours in restless apprehension waiting for Israel, my partner, to return from work at the end of the day. Israel was an essential worker at a medical cannabis facility; after debating our limited options with the limited information we had available to us, we had decided that they would continue working so our income would not be disrupted in a time of crisis. Having been away from Brazil, my home country, for over a decade, and having only immigrated to Canada from the US one year prior to the pandemic, I deeply feared financial hardship. My social support was limited, and we needed some financial cushion to be able to go through the immigration process and stay in Canada. Being a newcomer immigrant often means having to pay higher fees for everything, as personal and family credit history play a major role in what services are accessible to you.

Other than our immigrant status, our financial lives were similar to other millennials without generational wealth. We lived paycheck to paycheck, agonized over which bills to prioritize, and struggled to build savings. Despite our circumstances, for a long time, I deeply regretted having chosen to risk COVID exposure over financial loss. Thinking about it leaves a bitter taste in my mouth—the taste of injustice. Today, I accept that we were given no other option. But I will never forget the unjust choice we were forced to make between our basic income and our health. It's immoral and economically unsustainable, for individuals and for communities.

What started as a migraine quickly evolved to nausea, diarrhea, abdominal pain, chills, intense fatigue, and breathlessness. Lying on the couch and feeling like I had a grand piano on my chest, I decided to call telehealth. The nurse on the other side of the line immediately sent an ambulance to my home, because I was gasping for air while trying to say my name. It took three minutes for the paramedics to come, but it felt like an eternity. I started to say goodbye to my partner, through tears, as my brain swiped through all the possible outcomes of this situation. *Would I go to the hospital and never come back? How would Israel, who was also feeling terribly ill, fare alone at home?* I was so scared. But when the paramedics came, they told me to get tested and stay home. So, Israel and I got tested on our third day of symptoms. Testing was very limited, and we were only able to test because Israel was an essential worker. To our surprise, we tested negative.

But despite my negative result, I went on to develop myriad multi system symptoms that fluctuated in nature, number, severity, and duration, leaving me feeling confused and isolated. I was having a different experience from what the world was telling me COVID-19 looked like: an illness that would either kill or last only fourteen days—a fallacy, to say the least. One week after what was obviously a false negative, scared for our lives and struggling to care for ourselves at home, we decided to try to get tested again. But we were vehemently denied.

A false negative test results from failure to detect viral material in a sample from an infected individual; this is an intrinsic and expected feature of PCR tests, the only type of test that was available at the time. However, like many others without a positive PCR test (either due to false negative test results or limited access to testing), not having a confirmatory test result was held against us by health care providers, employers, and insurance providers, who saw it as the ultimate evidence to deny what our bodies were experiencing and invalidate our concerns. We were left with the burden of proving that we had been exposed, and that such exposure could be traced back to Israel's workplace. Thus, seeking worker's compensation through Ontario's Workplace Safety and Insurance Board was an experience of deep emotional distress and trauma. We were repeatedly told that we did not have COVID-19 because we lacked a positive PCR test.

Even when we got others to acknowledge we'd had COVID-19 at some point, we were treated with disbelief when it came to reporting long-term health problems associated with the initial illness. The case worker handling the process told us no one was sick with COVID for as long as we were, and that nobody was going to pay for us to stay home and do nothing. I sought to gather medical documentation, to prove that our long-term medical concerns were real and tied to COVID-19, but after every appointment, we were met with gaslighting and mediocre health care practices. The stress and mental exertion of advocating for ourselves to medical providers triggered episodes of PEM, with symptom relapses that left me bed-bound for weeks at a time. I quickly realized that seeking a diagnosis under these circumstances was often too costly for my health, and that the process required pacing and planning on my part to avoid worsening my overall health and well-being. It took us fourteen months to get a Long COVID diagnosis in our medical records. We were able to be diagnosed because

I connected with another patient on Instagram, who recommended a doctor in our area who was knowledgeable about Long COVID (for more on how to get a diagnosis, see chapter 6).

Unfortunately, and going against evidence-based reasoning, some employers and insurance providers still rely on proof of infection based on positive test results. Thus, a positive test can help you advocate for yourself with employers and insurance providers. But here's the caveat: In seeking a positive test result, consider the costs you may incur to your well-being and PEM management (if applicable), including your mental health. Take into account that the chance of false negatives is neither nil nor negligible for all COVID-19 diagnostic tests, document your symptoms as best you can (see page 123) and seek a clinical diagnosis, which can often carry the same weight as a positive test result.

To dodge gaslighting and medical violence through the deliberate delivery of suboptimal, insufficient, and inadequate care, your best chance of finding an informed health care provider who is willing to work with Long COVID patients is by talking with long-haulers in your community. Connect with patients in your area through social media and support groups (see the resources on page 278). You can connect with the Long COVID, ME/CFS, and chronically ill communities on social media using the hashtags #FBLC ("Follow Back Long COVID"), #pwLC (people with Long COVID), #pwME ("people with ME/CFS"), and #NEISVoid ("No End In Sight Void"), a tag created by disability advocate Brianne Bennes to connect a community that believes people first, refrains from unsolicited advice, and truly listens to the struggles of those with chronic illnesses.[4]

Find out how other long-haulers in your area are faring and who they are seeing. And keep in mind that Long COVID specialists and knowledgeable health professionals can be hard to come by. While policy, research, and clinical practice catches up, your community is your best and most compassionate resource.

In the months following the first COVID-19 symptoms, I became mostly bedridden, and my family's financial situation further eroded as the goal of returning to our previous health became a moving target. I was only able to maintain my job because of my workload and schedule flexibility, as well as my partner's ability to take care of our basic household needs so I could use my energy to produce an income. Household duties can be very difficult for someone with a chronic illness that involves PEM. Israel is now unable to perform their previous job duties because of PEM, persistent fatigue, chronic pain, and brain fog, among other health issues, and their only option has been unpaid medical leave. Even after a clinical diagnosis of Long COVID, Israel's employer leveraged a lack of evidence of contact tracing to repeatedly deny them work accommodations, arguing that there's no proof that they became infected at work.

As we searched for answers, it very quickly became clear to us that the current systems ostracize workers seeking help and overwhelmingly benefit the employer, while rejecting evidence-based reasoning that both testing and tracing are intrinsically imperfect. After talking to others in our patient support group, we came to the realization that reapplying for workers' compensation was not worth the health costs, given the current policies in place. If you find yourself in a similar situation, know that it is not a failure to stop pursuing avenues of support that have failed you.

Forced into hero status against our will, we were given a "thank you for your service" token and left to struggle alone. Our income was supplemented by the Canada Emergency Response Benefit (CERB), which meant we received a taxable amount of five hundred Canadian dollars per week for twenty-eight weeks. CERB simply was not sufficient to support even one chronically ill and disabled adult, let alone two. When our eligibility for CERB payments ended, our financial struggle escalated quickly. We had to negotiate the loan on our car and make agreements with utility companies, all of which fulfilled our immediate needs to get by, while furthering our long-term financial loss and draining the limited energy we might have used to care for ourselves.

Seventeen months after being awakened by my first COVID-19 symptom, my family was facing homelessness. We had no savings or enough income to survive. We were left with no other choice but to sell all of our belongings and relocate to Brazil, where the cost of living is lower and we would have access to the country's universal health system—which, although limited and underfunded, we felt would provide more accessible health care than the Canadian health care system.

Nearly two years into this illness, my quality of life has decreased substantially, partially because we don't have adequate access to the things we need to manage Long COVID symptoms—a situation directly tied to lack of financial resources. I'm now in the position of having to reassess a beloved career with a master's and a PhD that took me fourteen years to build; I've been forced to completely reimagine my professional identity with the limitations imposed by chronic illness. As I rely on resilience and constantly try to rebuild and adapt to life with Long COVID, I grapple with much rage. This anger comes from knowing that my family isn't alone in this experience; many people are financially struggling while chronically ill because they were forced to work for income during a pandemic, without systems in place to allow for rest and safety. Most of us who don't have the proof of a positive test are unable to access care and social support due to willful ignorance and denial regarding what COVID-19 and its aftermath can look like. Instead, we rely on the work and expertise of disability activists and chronically ill people to show us the way and give us the support that social systems should be providing.

No Help and No Plan: Thrust into the Shadow Pandemic of Post-Viral Illness

Karyn Bishof

I had a moderate, nonhospitalized case of COVID in March 2020, and I'm now a disabled long-hauler, still very sick. As a single mother, unable to work since April 2020, and limited to my bed 85 percent of the time, I'm out of options. I have seen firsthand that no financial assistance exists for those dealing with Long COVID and its associated conditions.

I contracted COVID-19 while working as a firefighter/paramedic in South Florida. At the time, I was very active; I played soccer and did high-intensity workouts five to six times a week. Getting COVID changed it all. I have seen forty doctors, participated in three studies, and received sixty diagnoses for conditions triggered by COVID-19. I still suffer over eighty-five symptoms. Even though I was a health care worker, before I got COVID-19 I never understood what living with chronic illness was really like, or how taxing it is to navigate the disability system or the medical gaslighting. Now, I realize.

I was rapidly thrust into the world of complex chronic illness. I had no choice but to quickly learn about the conditions occurring at very high rates within the Long COVID community, like POTS (postural orthostatic tachycardia syndrome), ME/CFS, MCAS (mast cell activation syndrome), fibromyalgia, NDPH (new daily persistent headache), migraines, SFN (small fiber neuropathy), IBS (irritable bowel syndrome), HSD (hypermobility spectrum disorder), insomnia, autoimmune diseases, and more. These conditions leave many of us debilitated, stuck in bed, unable to work or function in everyday life—I know, because I have been diagnosed with several of these illnesses. Many of them lack research, specialists, and funding. This results in substantial medical gaslighting, which I have unfortunately become all too familiar with. But no matter how often it happens, I'm still not numb to it. Being disbelieved by providers, case workers, and insurance companies hurts just as much, every time it happens. Years into the pandemic, we are still experiencing gaslighting.

I was terminated in April 2020. In May 2020, I sought medical care for the first time since becoming sick, when I started to experience new symptoms that I didn't have during my acute infection and previous symptoms that had gone away or decreased came back with a vengeance. Workers' compensation sent me to urgent care, where health care providers assured me I was "fine" because my lungs were clear. Of course, no one knew about Long COVID at that time. In June, workers' compensation denied my claim because my employer countered my claim that I'd been infected on the job. I had to work to prove that my employer had lied to get my benefits reinstated. Only three months into my illness, it was already clear to me that long-haulers would face many barriers to care, starting with credibility and financial support. As one of the first people going through it, I knew I had to connect with others and try to share what I'd learned. In late June 2020, I created the COVID-19 Longhauler Advocacy Project (C-19 LAP), which focuses on advocacy, education research, and support for long-haulers, medical professionals, and researchers studying the disease. Part of its purpose was to unite long-haulers and raise awareness about Long COVID—which we have succeeded in doing. But there's still a lot more work to do.

In November 2020, I was sent to another workers' compensation doctor. I brought my scrupulously documented medical records, because I figured the more "proof" I could provide of my illness, the more seriously I'd be taken. I was wrong. The doctor denied my benefits. Even worse, she wrote in my file that the fact that I had brought along my binder with medical records suggested I had a mental illness. After that, no more benefits came from workers' compensation.

As a long-hauler, there is no magic formula that will make health care providers believe you. If you don't document your illness, you lack proof. If you do, you must be crazy. There's nothing I could have done that day to guarantee belief from a doctor who was clearly skeptical, but if I could go back in time and talk to myself then, I'd warn myself that some doctors have fragile egos. I'd tell myself that, while my ability to be organized, competent and diligent has gotten me most things in life I deserve, in this situation, it might work against me.

Over the next year, unemployment helped me survive—barely—but in May 2021, Florida's governor decided not to renew federal assistance programs. Instead, he reinstated "work search" requirements for unemployment benefits, causing thousands of long-haulers—like me—to become ineligible. I couldn't search for work, because I couldn't work. Like many other chronically ill and disabled people, my only option was accepting poverty. April 2021 was the last time I received any type of "income" other than the whopping $158 a month I get now via the Temporary Cash Assistance program from the Florida Department of Children and Families. Every month, I have to decide whether this money will go to paying my utility bills or for my medications.

After running out of options through unemployment and workers' compensation, and being completely unable to work, I applied for Social Security Disability Insurance (SSDI) in late April 2021. The application process alone was intimidating and demoralizing. I applied for SSDI under ten disabling conditions. I have the most extensive testing and documentation of any long-hauler I know—after all, I've worked as an advocate for the past year, helping the NIH to design studies and creating a Comprehensive Guide for COVID-19 Long-Haulers and Providers (see page 280). I've listened to and learned from others' experiences and expertise and even hosted a disability webinar for long-haulers. But even I was denied SSDI. Apparently, my case reviewers believe I can still work in some capacity.

I knew if I got denied, every long-hauler behind me was going to get denied, too. It made me sick to my stomach, and my thoughts spiraled. *What am I going to do? How am I going to pay my bills, afford my medications, or put gas in my car to get to my doctors?* It's a 24-7 constant dread and worry that drastically and adversely impacts my health and "recovery." What concerns me even more is that no one—outside of the long-hauler community—is creating financial assistance for long-haulers. In November 2021, I submitted my appeal for SSDI; in March 2022, I was denied again. As of this writing, my next step is to move on to a hearing. But even if I qualify for SSDI this time around, I'll still be in a dire financial position. SSDI monthly payments are low—the average SSDI benefit per month in January 2022 was $1,358.50.[5]

The options that currently exist aren't sufficient, and many people aren't even eligible for them to begin with. Most of us have exhausted all of our options, and programs like pandemic unemployment and stimulus checks have ended. Through my organization C-19 LAP, we have been working to raise awareness about and help expedite programs that can provide assistance to long-haulers. In January 2022, we sent a letter to US government leaders about the long-term financial implications—both to individuals and the economy—of Long COVID and, as of this writing, we are working with several members of Congress to push for Long COVID assistance programs and a Long COVID task force. We helped draft Representative Ayanna Pressley's Treat Long Covid Act in April, and we have met with the White House COVID-19 Response Team, Health and Human Services, and the Department of Labor to further our efforts. The most important goal for us is mandatory, meaningful patient engagement at each step of the process. We are adamantly trying to ensure Long COVID patients have a seat at the table and input in their futures.

Long COVID patients have become experts. From the very early months of the pandemic, we have taken on the roles of researchers, advocates, journalists, educators, community support leaders, and more. Other chronic illness communities have shared their knowledge, and this guidance has made us the strong, driven, knowledgeable advocates we are today; we stop at nothing to ensure millions receive help. For many, these opportunities will unfortunately not come soon enough.

What do we do in the meantime? We can't pay our bills, we've gone into extreme debt, we can't afford our medications, and some of us have been left homeless. The stress of our financial losses is overwhelming. None of us want to be sick, disabled, or unable to participate in our own daily lives. None of us want to be dependent on someone else, let alone the government. We are desperate for answers and for help, but it will take years and potentially decades until research is completed and treatments are found. We have no choice but to depend on a system that was already broken and is clearly incapable of handling the mass influx of millions of long-haulers applying for disability. Even as we depend on these systems and try to make them work for us, we can and should still fight for better solutions. In advocacy, I found an outlet for my own frustrations and a way to learn about myself and my condition while connecting with and helping others in my situation. Maybe you will do the same. We must overhaul the disability system, so it not only more readily and easily accepts people, but also provides assistance that we can actually survive off of.

Navigating the system as a disabled person is hard and can take a long time. However, there are resources and organizations out there working to make this process easier and more inclusive. It's important that you utilize these resources and then apply what you learn to your own care, case, and needs.

Practical Tips for Navigating Financial Struggles with Energy-Limiting Chronic Illness

Alison Sbrana

In 2014, I got a virus and never recovered. Now, I live with ME/CFS. At the beginning of the pandemic, I and many others in the ME/CFS community feared that COVID-19 would cause post-viral illness, because so many of us had developed chronic illnesses following an infection. Because of my professional background as a case manager and my personal lived experience with viral-triggered ME/CFS, I worried that people experiencing chronic illness after COVID would have a difficult path of financial struggle, employment difficulties, and barriers accessing disability benefits ahead of them. In May 2020, I got involved with Long COVID advocacy, to help long-haulers navigate these challenges. The first piece of advice I give to people with Long COVID is this: You have a disability now. There are disability rights and benefits that exist to help protect you at your job and provide you with benefits if you can't work, and there is a large community of disabled people here to help you navigate them. These resources are not perfect by any means—and a community of advocates works every day to improve them—but the sooner you understand this, the easier it will be to support your body and its new needs as you learn to live with Long COVID.

I didn't know I was disabled until several years into my illness. I had false perceptions of what disability looked like due to stereotypes (I didn't understand that a dynamic, fluctuating health condition could and often does fit the definition of disability), so even though I was aware that disability rights and benefits existed, I didn't understand that I could benefit from them. I went through years of pushing myself and crashing while job-hopping, in a desperate attempt to find employment that would work for an unpredictable, fluctuating chronic illness—without requesting accommodations. These efforts were not successful and led to worse health outcomes for me.

So, here I am, telling you what I wish someone had told me.

Navigating employment and financial hardships while living with an unpredictable, fluctuating chronic illness like Long COVID is an extremely difficult task. So, you need to ask for help from organizations and disability advocates who have experience in this area. I'll start by telling you what I know. Disclaimer: My area of expertise is in benefits and programs within the US; if you are outside of the US, you can likely receive more specific advice by asking for referrals from local disability advocates or groups in your area.

I. DRAW ON DISABLED COMMUNITY TIPS TO SURVIVE FINANCIALLY

It's difficult to survive financially with an unpredictable and fluctuating illness like Long COVID, especially when government safety nets are inadequate.

First, as we stated at the beginning of this chapter, this is not your fault. It's not your fault that you have Long COVID. It's not your fault that there are no adequate financial safety nets to support people while they recover or experience ongoing symptoms after COVID-19. It's not a personal failure if you ran out of savings and are struggling to get by. It's not your fault if you're in debt trying to pay for basic needs, if you lose your house, or if you lose your car. It's a systemic failure. Remind yourself of this on days when money is tight and you're making tough choices about what and where to spend.

The second thing I want you to know is that you're not alone in your financial struggle. Remember, this is a system failure, which means many other people are in the same boat. People with chronic illnesses and disabilities have struggled financially for many years before the pandemic. The good news (unfortunately) is this means we have a community to help us navigate this struggle; there is wisdom from disabled elders to help guide us.

One of the best examples I know of this is the How to Get On website, a WordPress blog, created to help people with chronic illness (especially ME/CFS) self-advocate for government assistance, disability benefits, and more. If finances are a concern for you, go to HowToGetOn.wordpress.com and bookmark the site. An entire section of the website is dedicated to financial survival and addresses how to navigate various programs that help with the financial burden of chronic illnesses like Long COVID.

2. EDUCATE YOURSELF ABOUT DISABILITY BENEFITS

The first thing to know when applying for disability benefits or workers' compensation is that this system rarely adequately helps disabled people, and many people are unfairly denied benefits. Benefits like disability insurance were created within systems where ableism, sexism, homophobia, racism, and other forms of institutionalized violence exist, so they can be difficult to access, especially for people facing overlapping sources of oppression. It's natural and common to take it personally when you get a denial letter or struggle to access benefits, but you will not be alone in this experience, and waiting to apply out of fear or intimidation can delay your benefits. I myself waited far too long to apply, after hearing horror stories, but I was actually approved for Social Security Disability Insurance on my first try. This is not going to be the case for everyone (as we know from Karyn's story)—statistics from 2008 to 2017 show between a 20 to 25 percent approval rate for initial applications—but it can happen.

If you're denied disability benefits or workers' compensation, it's not your fault, nor is it a reflection of how disabled or sick you are. It's a system failure. Please don't let the denial letters intimidate you into giving up. It is not uncommon for people who are initially denied benefits to be able to access them eventually via the appeals process. There is a time window for appeals, so when you get that first denial letter, you need to be prepared and act quickly to find a lawyer who fits your needs and can take your appeal on if you don't have one already.

When looking for a lawyer, look for one who specifically works on the benefit type you are navigating; some lawyers specialize in Social Security, others work on short- and long-term disability insurance you access through work, and so on. Ask your Center for Independent Living or a state- or region-wide disability advocacy organization for recommendations if you can. Seeking legal advice can feel intimidating and expensive, especially at a time when finances are limited. However, it's important to consider legal help, because you risk losing out on thousands of dollars of benefits. Oftentimes lawyers will work on contingency, meaning they are only paid if they win your case and their compensation comes out of your backpay, so you don't have to pay legal fees upfront at a time when you have very limited resources.

Remember that you paid into these benefits—whether they are private benefits your workplace paid for with a disability insurance policy or Social Security funded by your tax dollars—and you deserve to access them if Long COVID makes it difficult for you to work or causes symptom exacerbation on a regular or frequent basis that interferes with your life.

There are many complexities to disability benefits and workers' compensation. That's why it's so important to consult with someone in your area—whether at your local Center for Independent Living, with a case manager or social worker at your health care provider's office or elsewhere, or with a disability lawyer—to talk about options for your individual circumstances.

3. ASK FOR ACCOMMODATIONS AT WORK

Long COVID can be considered a disability under civil rights laws in the US, including the Americans with Disabilities Act (ADA). The ADA is the 1990 civil rights law protecting people with disabilities from discrimination and giving them equal opportunity to participate in life activities, including employment. The Federal Office for Civil Rights published a six-page handout titled *Guidance on "Long COVID" as a Disability Under the ADA, Section 504, and Section 1557* (see page 279). I encourage you to search for this online, as it explains specifically how Long COVID can be a disability under civil rights laws and what your rights are under those laws, using a simple question-and-answer format with bullet points providing examples.

If you're specifically seeking help with accommodations at work, the Job Accommodations Network is funded by the Department of Labor Office of Disability Employment Policy to help with this. Their website, askjan.org, is a great resource to learn more about the accommodations process and your rights under the ADA. Askjan.org also has excellent resources specifically tailored to Long COVID, including suggested accommodations based on Long COVID symptoms. If you want more personalized advice, you can also talk to them directly for an individualized consultation. This can be done via phone at (800) 526-7234 (Voice) or (877) 781-9403 (TTY), or you can fill out the *JAN on Demand* form on their website for an email consult.

4. APPLY FOR GOVERNMENT ASSISTANCE

Government assistance programs can help reduce expenses, which is important when disability benefits don't cover all of your expenses. The average Social Security Disability Insurance benefit *per month* in January 2022 was $1,358.50[6]—in short, you won't get one all-encompassing cash benefit that covers all of your expenses, so you'll need to stretch your budget further by using these programs. Benefits vary widely between states, so it's important to talk to someone in your state who can help you identify which programs you might qualify for. Talk to your Center for Independent Living or ask your health care provider to refer you to a social worker or case manager to help you. If you would benefit from help with daily tasks like bathing and meals—even if a family member is currently providing that help—I encourage you to search for your local Aging and Disability Resource Center (ADRC) and reach out. ADRCs are government offices that help people understand options for help at home with tasks like showering safely, getting dressed (including compression stockings for those with POTS), medication management, meal preparation, and getting around your home and community safely.

Don't be intimidated by the word *disability* here—if you are struggling with tasks like these, please reach out to your local office. I personally receive these services through my state's Medicaid program; they have improved my quality of life substantially. For example, while I only receive about $1,100 per month from SSDI, I am allocated a budget of about $3,000 per month for help with personal care, homemaking, and medical tasks through a fiscal management agency for Home and Community Based Services with Medicaid in my state. This money is for help with tasks like picking up my prescriptions, making sure I'm safe while showering with POTS, doing laundry, going to the grocery store, and preparing meals. My spouse is one of my paid caregivers, because he knows the specifics of how to help my symptoms and accommodate me. These services were much easier for me to access than SSDI. However, my ease of access was in large part due to the expanded Medicaid program in my state, which includes an excellent disability buy-in program; services do vary significantly from state to state, because Medicaid (and the Home and Community Based Services it provides) is a state-run program whereas SSDI is federal, and the application process can be lengthy.

5. SEEK HELP WITH HEALTH INSURANCE AND MEDICAL BILLS

Government assistance programs for health insurance and medical benefits can be essential to financial (and literal) survival when you live with a chronic condition in the US. Health insurance options are complex, so the most important advice here is to find a local expert by going to localhelp.healthcare.gov to find a professional health coverage guide or enrollment assister near you and make an appointment. I did this when I was struggling to maintain employment due to my symptoms in my third year of being sick, and I learned about a program in my state that helps people with disabilities get access to Medicaid without restrictive income or asset limits. That program changed my life, because I was guaranteed health insurance even if I couldn't work anymore.

Hospitals often have charity care or financial assistance that you may qualify for, so ask about that before you pay a hospital bill. I applied for a statewide financial assistance program, with help from a billing specialist at my local federally qualified health center, so I could get iron infusions, and it brought my bill from over six thousand dollars to less than two hundred. If you've exhausted all options for reducing your bill and still intend to pay, payment plans may also be available, so call the number on your bill and ask about that, especially before putting a medical bill on a credit card, which will typically have higher interest than a payment plan offered by a medical office.

If you are having difficulty finding any of the offices listed above near you, please call United Way's 211 or use their online web service. You will definitely want help applying for government assistance from someone like a social worker, case manager, or enrollment assister for Medicaid or subsidized Marketplace health insurance plans, as government benefits can be confusing, and it's helpful to have a direct contact if issues arise with your benefits.

6. UTILIZE LOCAL HELP THROUGH CENTERS FOR INDEPENDENT LIVING

It's a good idea to seek local help when navigating financial and employment issues related to Long COVID, as government assistance and local resources vary widely based on location. Centers for Independent Living (CIL) are community-based nonprofits run by people with disabilities to help people with disabilities. To find a location near you, go to the Administration for Community Living website at ACL.gov. Your CIL can help you by connecting you with tools, resources, and support to make your new normal living with Long COVID a little easier. Each CIL differs, so reach out to your local office to inquire about how they can help you.

The CIL in my area assigned me a case worker who helped me understand that I could apply for SSDI—and that, once approved, I could even work part-time, which brought me hope for my future. She helped me with my application for Social Security Disability Insurance in a way that accommodated my fatigue and post-exertional malaise. Having someone who understood the disability benefits system and who also was disabled herself helped me feel comfortable and not as intimidated by the questions.

It can be difficult to adjust to a new normal with Long COVID, especially when financial worries and benefits denials can be daily stressors. But there is a community of disabled and chronically ill folks who have been down this difficult path before you, and I hope the wisdom we have gained from our lived experiences makes this process a little easier for you, especially while activists work on paving a new path to help future generations of chronically ill and disabled folks. Please do ask for help from the resources mentioned above, and don't wait for any provider, employer, or other official to use the word *disability* to do so. The existing assistance programs, disability benefits, and legal protections aren't perfect by any means, but they do make life a little easier. When you're living with an illness that is poorly understood with minimal options for treatment, that added ease can really make a difference. It sure has for me.

Each of our journeys through chronic illness, disability, and financial struggle have been uneven—with some highs and many lows. Our strength lies in the knowledge of our community and the stories of those, like us, who have gone through it already. If you find yourself in a similar situation, take solace in knowing that you are not alone in this experience. Struggling financially is not a personal failure, but rather a systemic issue.

All three of us have found support and resources within our patient community, and we encourage you to do the same. While resources and guidance may frequently change, there are some extraordinary patient-led Long COVID groups[7] doing a lot of work for the community. Utilize and join these communities, especially regional and local groups that can provide information on community-specific resources. Body Politic hosts a support group outside of social media on a platform called Slack. On Facebook, you can find the COVID-19 Longhauler Advocacy Project, which also has US state chapters and special population groups including pediatrics. You can connect with other Long COVID patients and activists in Canada through the COVID Long-Haulers Canada group on Facebook, which includes provincial level chapters.

Many generations of disability activists have been advocating for new and improved policies to assist disabled people. There is a legion of chronic illness and disability activists fighting to improve the lives and financial stability of people living with Long COVID. You, too, can join our ranks to fight for change.

Survival Tips

It's not your fault that you have Long COVID. When it comes to financial survival, know that it's not a personal failure if you run out of savings and are struggling to get by, if you're in debt trying to pay for basic needs, or if you lose your house or car because you can't keep up with payments.

To help you cope with these challenges, there are disability rights that can help protect you at your job, assistance programs that can help if you can't work enough to support yourself, and there's a community of disabled people who can help you navigate these rights and programs. These rights and benefits aren't easy to navigate nor are they set up to be fair or equitable, so to get support accessing them we recommend you do the following:

- Draw on disabled-community tips to survive financially, including from patient-led Long COVID support groups in your country and local area, as well as resources from well-established disability communities like HowToGetOn.wordpress.com.

- Ask for accommodations at work using the website AskJan.org to help you. It has suggested accommodations for common Long COVID symptoms and information about the process of requesting reasonable accommodations.

- Ask for help from the Centers for Independent Living (CIL) in your area.

- Apply for government assistance using local help from your local CIL, from a case manager or social worker at your health care provider's office, or by calling 211 (United Way's local resource referral program). If you need help with tasks at home, contact your local Aging and Disability Resource Center (ADRC).

- For health insurance, find a local enrollment assister at localhelp. healthcare.gov to help you understand what health insurance programs or financial assistance you might qualify for. For hospital bills, check to see if you qualify for charity care programs. Call the number on your medical bill to discuss payment plans and financial assistance options.

- Seek legal advice promptly if you are denied disability benefits to help with your appeal. Consider seeking legal advice for the initial application to help increase your chance of approval. When finding a lawyer, ask for recommendations from disability organizations in your area, and make sure to be mindful of the type of benefits lawyer you need based on what you are applying for.

Closer Than They Seem

Finding a Caregiver

Chimére L. Smith

March 22, 2020

Dear Self,

You are a wonderful woman whose widened wings will not waste or wither under the wayward weight of this war-torn world. You will overcome the uncertainty of Corona by reaching out to loved ones, helping those in need, and relaxing in a place of power and peace.

You are going to take amazing care of yourself, and you are shifting into the shiftless softness of sacred sanity.

You are well within your right to chill, sleep, write, and walk as you please.

You deserve this. I am prepared for this moment.

The journal entry I wrote on the day I will never forget was full of flowery hopes and dreams of what my life during a pandemic would become. It all sounded so magical and—dare I say—possible. As an exhausted teacher and undisclosed introvert, I was starving for this time away from students, parents, and even friends and loved ones. Having Maryland's governor, Larry Hogan, declare a state of emergency that would close all schools for two weeks was an unexpected gift I sorely needed—or so it seemed.

Yet, an explosive amount of alliteration covered up a tiny secret. My throat was catching fire as if doused in gasoline. Every few minutes while writing, I would stop to cough a little to clear it. I was so intent on making my journal entry as optimistic as possible that I tried to quell the question that grew in the pit of my belly. "Why was my throat hurting so badly when I had just gotten over a little bug two weeks ago?"

For the last two years, I have read this entry so often that I could probably recite it, if forced. Usually, my eyes are brimming with tears as I wonder if I have ever lied to myself more. With a shaky hand, I wrote this bullshit to try to convince myself I could withstand the weight of a pandemic.

Somehow, I knew I couldn't.

Reading the journal entry, I know those aren't my words. The entry was an act of deliberate pretense I had grown accustomed to delivering. Like Leonardo

DiCaprio's character in *Catch Me If You Can*, if I was going to document the last day before the end, I was going to make it as shimmery and magical as possible—even if it was all a big, fat-ass lie. No, I wasn't some psychopathic con artist. I had just gotten very good at lying to myself to make everyone else's world comfortable while my own was falling apart—even in my journal. I vomited this written garbage while my relationship with the man I loved more than anything was falling apart, while my throat burned, and while the anxiety I tried to ignore painted pictures foreshadowing what would happen to me and others during the pandemic. Writing the world's phoniest set of intentions and affirmations helped to dull these unspoken fears.

Later, I would wonder if maybe I caused this to happen to me—the sore throat, the broken relationship, and the damning future that would have me crawling from a bed to a toilet to a shower at the speed of the world's most inept tortoise for over a year. Only Steven Spielberg or M. Night Shyamalan could have written characters and events so catastrophically terrifying. But I would fare far worse than any scene from a scary movie.

Looking back, I somehow knew my throat was the first sign of my demise, but it would not be the last. Recalling all the COVID news stories and broadcasts I obsessed over, I didn't remember reading about anyone complaining of a sore throat or fatigue, and no doctors, who spoke on what seemed to be endangering only a small number of Americans at the time, mentioned this as a symptom. On some deep level, I just knew to expect the worst, which meant paying close attention to how my body slumped over in exhaustion as I wrote those dishonest words, how my eyes watered despite no apparent allergic reaction, and the way my boyfriend, Anthony's, bedroom spun as I entered it to sleep.

My God, I knew from the very first moment that I had it. Lying to a journal would never change that.

I just knew.

I didn't need anyone for shit. I'm a Black woman. The word *need* simply didn't exist in my vocabulary.

Black women *want, desire, crave, seek, shift, survive,* and *accomplish.* But we often make it our mission to never ever need a motherfucker for anything. The world teaches us this crucial lesson from birth. We learn it the first time our parents disappoint or leave us. The moment our hearts are shattered after that first heartbreak. The very first time we are fed poisonous rhetoric about why a white person got the call, job, or opportunity instead of us—when we are better qualified. It is emblazoned in our minds and hearts so clearly. We do whatever possible to assure ourselves that needing people is like shit—a substance that only belongs in the toilet to be flushed.

I have never had to explain to another Black woman why needing anyone is the Devil's work. We stir the knowledge of this mantra in our coffee and use it to season the food on our plates. And even though no one has ever found it, it is a Scripture in the Bibles we carry to church. I hear the revoking of need in our conversations. Read the disdain for it in between lines in text messages. I can smell it on our skin—mingling with the finest perfumes—when we gather in rooms to discuss almost anything.

Needing anything or anyone was the enemy. Expressing that need would invoke a national security threat. And what Black woman has time for all of that?

Needing is too lazy, vulnerable, sketchy, and inconsistent for us. To express a need of any kind would be admitting that our flagrant, cultured, creative tongues and ideas aren't as powerful as we want to believe. It would destroy our ecosystems full of people and entities that rely on us to keep up the sordid act, to do what needs to be done, to give what needs to be given.

Need—since becoming a teacher in 2015, I had done everything possible to assure that the word hardly ever crossed my lips. When I took a job working with middle school students in Baltimore City, I was sure of one thing: I would never ever need anyone again. I'd spent five years as a makeup artist, living paycheck to paycheck, borrowing money from family members and friends more times than I could count. At thirty-two, teaching was the perfect career move for me. I had an English degree, a penchant for writing, and an obsession with good grammar. While the local news painted the city's schools as failing and corrupt, I knew I would excel because I was a product of similar schools. If I could make it in a Baltimore school, I could make it anywhere.

Receiving my first check made me squeal with joy. It was enough to pay every bill, and left me with additional money to do what I wanted two times over. I didn't even have to take on any more makeup clients if I didn't want to. Who cared that teachers were still the lowest paid professionals in America, doing more work than most? For a woman who grew up in the projects of Washington, DC, I was "hood rich" and damn proud of myself.

I don't believe I feared being sick or even dying as much as I feared having to ask others for support. The thought alone caused my bones to shake and my mind to go blank.

When I got COVID, I would not and could not share with anyone that I might be dying. I refused to call anyone to say that I needed medicine, rides to the hospitals, or the Pedialyte I struggled to swallow.

Stumbling from my first doctor and urgent care visits, I felt ashamed of myself for knowing I needed prayer from those I loved and held close. I was supposed to be at their epicenter, waiting to catch each of their needs and meet them. Yet, here I was, one step away from leeching off of them. So used to not having to extend my hand to accept much from anyone for so long, I tucked my desperation in the parts of my heart where I don't often go.

I asked for nothing, and I told no one of what coursed through my body. No one except Mom.

I'd heard of her months before I saw her. It was 2004 and Eric,* my then-boyfriend, told me how much he loved and adored her—Pastor Paula Murray. Eric attended a small church in Baltimore where she was the founding pastor and, one day, he told me he wanted us to go to a service together. I couldn't wait. At twenty-two years old, I knew that if a man wanted to take me to his church, he was hoping to make me a permanent part of his future.

We pulled up on a corner in a shady area with liquor stores and food spots with people lined up outside. I had lived in Baltimore for a year, but I'd never been to this part of town before. Turning my head to check my surroundings, I saw a green and white building with an awning and ramp. Nervous and excited, I pulled in closer to Eric as we walked toward Pilgrim Temple Church, Inc., as the sign read. Pastor Paula Murray's name was at the bottom. We were going to church on a Friday night!

We walked up to the building, and I heard the drums, the bass guitar, and the gravelly sound of a man's voice. Eric peered into the glass window of the door, a sign of respect that was a familiar gesture at many Black churches. If I knew

---

* Names of ex-boyfriends have been changed in this chapter.

anything growing up in a similar environment in Washington, DC, it was that we didn't just bust up in a church without checking the scene first. It was an unspoken rule that we were not to enter while someone was praying, prophesying, or preaching, without being given permission.

We were safe to enter "The Temple," as I had heard him call it many times before. The sanctuary was intimate and inviting. Every pew was filled, but some members made space for us near the middle. When my heart settled, my eyes led me to a short man with glasses and salt-and-pepper hair who instructed someone in the congregation to stand as he prepared to give them a "word"—a spiritual, prophetic message that preachers believe was given to them by God to help people understand the plans that are destined for their lives. Outside of the church, people like this are psychics or tarot readers. Some people believe that these types of services are a farce or a chance for self-proclaimed preachers to make money off of people's fear and faith. But, even as a child, I had always trusted that if someone said God gave them a message, then who was I to deny it?

The service closed with final remarks from a woman who barely reached the microphone on the pulpit. She wore a bus operating uniform and white footie socks with no shoes. My heart connected to the unique power in her voice immediately: It was husky and matter of fact. This was Pastor Paula Murray. She moved and swayed like a Southern Baptist preacher woman with a city flair. Her back was straight, and she was assured as she thanked her congregants and the prophet for coming out on a Friday night. There weren't many women pastors who led Black churches, so I knew she was something special. I knew she had taken risks to start her own church. Any woman with that much chutzpah, I wanted to meet.

Eric led me to Pastor Murray as she hugged the last churchgoers leaving the building. She was warm but stern, and she didn't seem to be the least bit impressed with me. She told me it was a pleasure to meet me and to make sure I returned for a Sunday church service. And so I did.

Two years later, Eric and I suffered a nasty breakup. It was the stuff of legends. I wanted to quit the church and everything associated with him. I was on the choir, the praise team, and the hospitality ministry, but I didn't care. I wanted out. When I presented my decision to Pastor Murray, she refused to accept it. She showered me with love, and told me to brush my shoulders off and pick myself up.

Seeing no way to argue with her, I stayed put, maintaining my position in the church and in her life. From that moment on, I stopped calling her Pastor Murray. Her advice and support was like that of a caring mother, and so without any fanfare, she became my "Mom" and Godmother; with my biological mother back in DC, Pastor Murray became my mother figure in Baltimore, the city where I chose to plant my roots as an adult.

In 2013, Mom had a room built for me in her home. I had been evicted from my apartment by the slumlord who owned it, causing me to strongly consider moving back to DC. When I cried to Mom about how much I loved Baltimore and didn't want to leave, I could tell she was about to do what she does so well: spring into action under pressure.

A week later, Mom invited me to bring all of my belongings to her house so I could stay in my new room. She and her eldest brother had brainstormed how to construct a room in her basement that would suit me perfectly. I don't know how many trips they made to Home Depot and Lowe's to erect walls, electrical outlets, and a door, but when I walked into that room, it felt like home.

I was finally home with my Mom.

Mom was no longer just my spiritual leader. She would pray for me when I experienced any hardship or setback and coddle me even when I was being spoiled and selfish; she was so proud of me whenever I accomplished any goal. No one was prouder of me for graduating from college and becoming a teacher than Mom. And if she thought for even a second that I was being mistreated, she would give that person a talkin' to so severe they would question her allegiance to the Lord.

She is one of the sweetest women I have ever met. One should never get it twisted: She is my ride or die. Mom was the first one to know how sick I truly was on that Wednesday in late March 2020, when I exhibited my first COVID-19 symptoms.

I don't know what made me decide to leave my then-boyfriend's house to come home to Mom three days after noticing my sore throat. Or maybe I do. Anthony refused to believe I was sick enough to warrant medical attention. That's when I knew that continuing to argue about symptoms he couldn't see—fatigue so intense that staying awake was as challenging as competing in the Olympics and the searing, burning pain I'd felt course through my back right before we were about to have sex—would kill me. He had even agreed with the two doctors I visited who tried to convince me that I had a mild sinus infection that Flonase and antibiotics would fix.

I loved him, but there was an unspoken battle brewing between us that would cause him to leave me a month after I left his house for the last time. He loved me, but I sensed that he didn't have my back. He couldn't protect or care for me—so I fled.

All I knew was I just wanted Mom. I wanted to be where I knew she was, even if we couldn't be in the same room. I wanted to be in my room, downstairs, listening to her animated voice talking loudly on a phone call or her beautiful crooning of any gospel song that crept into her mind. She made me feel safe. Even if she didn't know what to do, she always just knew what to do.

Hoping that Mom was too tired to come downstairs to greet me as she usually did, I weakly unlocked the door to our home. If I had what I suspected but didn't dare say aloud, I couldn't risk her contracting it, too. Mom was in her early sixties, a leader at a church, a mother, a grandmother, and a great-grandmother of two handsome young boys. She was a mover and shaker, putting to shame women half her age. I would have rather died than expose her, so I made sure to wear my mask as I hurried downstairs to my room.

Lead and steel were lighter than my body that first week. Sleep never came so easily. I didn't crave water or food. I just drowned in the sea that was my bed, begging for relief from what had surely come to kill me. At night, the darkness greeted me with sneering panic attacks that made me race around the basement, praying to God that whatever was chasing me would stop. Naked and drenched in sweat, I ran myself into a dizzying puddle on my bed, where sleep would lock me into her grip again, threatening to make my stay permanent.

I knew I had it.

The nights were also when my breathing became the most difficult. Lying down signaled The Coughing Committee to join at my bedside for our unscheduled meetings. I coughed so long and often that I don't know how I didn't meet my lungs in person. My throat was raw and scratchy, yet I wanted no water.

I didn't trust my body, which in a matter of days turned into 205 pounds of lucid nothingness, but I needed to put my faith in a God I could see. Though my arms, legs, hips, fingers, and ankles were in immense pain, I developed a skill my

Baptist history would scorn: praying without using words. My eyes closed as I imagined what I needed to pull from the recesses of my mind. My thoughts often landed on images of the hospital where I had gone each time I had caught some annoying little bug from one of my middle school students. I knew it would be crowded, but I silently prayed they would help me once again.

I felt relief when I remembered the hospital's kind staff, their smiling faces when they were on the verge of releasing me with a prescription for pink eye or the flu, and how close they were to my home. They would surely take care of me. They knew me. They knew my insurance card.

Sadly, they didn't take care of me this time. The workers barely even acknowledged me. Blue surgical masks hid the smiles of the nurses and doctors who were once so familiar. Ever since I was old enough to decide my own career path, I had always been told that a Black woman needed a job that offered good health insurance—even more than she needed a great salary. I had achieved that goal. But my trusty blue and white insurance card didn't matter to the front desk's reception. They looked past me and it. I still had to wait hours and hours to receive care. And the care I did not receive nearly killed me.

I would venture to this hospital—which became an intricate part of my private hell—at least six times over the course of the next six months. Every time, the health care providers I saw refused to acknowledge many of my symptoms. Outside of my triage room, I overheard doctors speaking about me, exchanging thoughts on some mystery infection they believed I had, while telling me to my face that I was healthy enough to be discharged. And when I confronted their administrative offices about my treatment, the staff blatantly ignored my concerns and complaints.

With or without words in my prayers, this was the first time I truly wondered, "Did God bother to hear me?"

Over time, I concocted what I believed to be a fail-safe plan for my now-regular hospital visits. I would wait until a little before dawn to leave the house to drive myself to the hospital. I was sure fewer people would be there in the wee hours of the morning. If I had to choose a time to die, it would be when there were fewer bodies commingling near mine, so I might be more easily identifiable. Fearing I wouldn't make it back home, but not wanting to worry Mom too much, I left notes for her at the bottom of the stairs letting her know which hospital I was headed to. On one of the notes, I included the names and numbers of people she should call if I passed away. In later months, I would chuckle as I remembered that she knew many of those people herself, so giving her their contact information was unnecessary. On the other hand, I understand my actions: Death knocked too loudly at my door too regularly for me to fail to take any precautions or allow for potential additional missteps.

Every time I made that trip to the hospital, I would will my hands to shift my Chevy's gears. Strength was the one thing I needed the most when I took those drives, but it was also the thing that never seemed to show up for me. How I made it to the hospital six times in six months without wrecking my car or killing someone else, I will never know. My eyes were always blurry. My mind was usually a blank cascade of nothingness. Heart racing, I hoped I would make it there fast enough to lie down on a lonely hospital bed. Wanting to die in the calmest, most dignified way became a goal of mine. Yet, there was not an ounce of dignity in how I was treated by the doctors who took hours to come to incredulously inquire about my condition. What I experienced felt worse than being turned away completely. I was left in cold, dark, and dank emergency rooms—alone—with no one to hold my hand to usher me into the bliss of the afterlife, should it come for me. I don't know if I would have ventured to the hospital so many times had I not been afraid of Mom finding my listless body in my bed in her basement.

After my initial infection, doctors and nurses refused me tests for two weeks. But I knew I had it, and so did they. They looked into my eyes, which were quickly turning yellowish red, with such pity and fear, sharing the frightening realization that we all could not speak. A nurse at the hospital near my home said, "We can't test you, but if you do have it, don't worry. You'll be just fine and back to normal in two weeks." Today, hearing the phrase "two weeks" in any conversation sends me into a tailspin that saps away the little energy I have left. My two weeks of acute illness followed by a breezy recovery never came. I knew they were lying. They never stopped lying. I never believed them.

Shortly after I left Anthony's house to come back to Mom's, I had stopped coming upstairs for anything except to walk out the front door to head to the hospital. I was mostly reduced to my room in the basement. Each step of the stairs leading to our living room and kitchen was a single mountain I couldn't even imagine myself climbing. While Mom made arrangements for the church to transition to virtual services, I stayed under enough blankets to warm a tiny city. Cradled in the darkness, I hoped she wouldn't even remember to call for me. Yet, I prayed that she would say something to assure me that I was still alive.

A few days into settling back at home with Mom, as I was sweating through chills, a fever, and a head heavier than the largest bowling ball I had ever held, my ears pricked up when I heard her call down, "Shug, what have you been eating and drinking down there? You haven't been up in a few days. Are you hungry?"

"No," I managed.

"Oh, well you gotta eat."

"I'm not hungry."

"OK."

With the doubtful inflection of those two letters along with the smell of bread toasting, I knew Mom was unfazed by my rejection of food or a beverage. She did what most mothers would—went into Super Mommy mode, packing her beloved Baltimore Ravens food tray with oatmeal, boiled eggs, a fruit cup, bottled water, and a cup of tea and placing it at the top of the stairs for me. She never shared that tray with anyone, so her placing it at the top of those stairs for me meant that she didn't care about possessions; she wanted me to eat to get well.

To Mom, I wasn't a patient, record, number, or statistic. I wasn't even Chimére. "Shug" was the name she had given me when I first moved in. It often amuses me when I consider how it so easily stuck to me. Shug Avery was the controversial antagonist turned beloved family friend in *The Color Purple*. We couldn't be less alike except that like Celie, Shug's friend and eventual caretaker, Mom had welcomed me into her life among her family—church and biological—daring anyone to dispute my place. It's a nickname I never wanted to change. I'm Chimmy, ChimChim, Chi, or Smizzle to others. But I'll always be Mom's Shug.

For about nine months, Mom and I primarily communicated via text. She would send me Scriptures and encouragement in short sentences. With her living on the top floor of our three-story home, she understood that my being so weak coupled with her bad knees made texting the only feasible way we could communicate.

One Sunday in March 2021, a year after I'd moved back in with her, Mom arrived home from church to see me in real clothes—a top and leggings. "Shug, you lookin' good with all the weight," she chuckled. I knew what that meant. All of the food she had cooked and forced me to eat at the height of my illness—along with the DoorDash deliveries of McDonald's Big Macs and fries—had come in handy. I was finally back to my pre-COVID weight, with some extra pounds sitting in all the right places.

Good mothers have a way of thinking (and actually saying) the most amusing and genuine things to show they see—really see—their children. They know how to sing the sneakiest prose of love. Mom noticing my body changing in a more positive way meant something to me. I believed her, and I wore my fluff with pride.

On the first day of November 2021, I said a teary-eyed goodbye to my room, the one Mom had made just for me. I moved into my own apartment.

Throughout the pandemic, I had felt a huge wave of maturity and evolution slamming into every area of my life. It was so strong that it threatened to drown me if I didn't ride the current. Each week, I looked around the space I had considered my sanctuary for eight years, knowing—with the kind of confidence that develops when we conquer trials that seem insurmountable and destructive—that I could no longer build my life around that tiny space. But a whole lot happened before I was able to make that move.

In April 2020, I started telling my story of courage, hope, and devastation to whoever would listen. I sent emails to doctors, hospital administrative teams, journalists, and politicians. Living with fear but willing to push on as if it didn't exist, I stopped accepting doctors' answers as law. And I started asking critical questions, ones that didn't just solve the mystery of how to save my own life but considered the plight of other Black Americans who suffered with Long COVID. I've probably talked to every media platform known to man. And my loud mouth ignited people from every corner of the world, rewarding me with gifts and cards of love and care. They peppered every nook of the room, so much that the space I once treasured more than anywhere else in the world started to feel too small for me.

In the face of exceptional adversity, I was forced to become a giant—in control of every dream, goal, and achievement meant for me. Eventually, thanks to Mom's thoughtful and constant care, I also began to learn how to better manage some of my symptoms, see small improvements in my health, and slowly become more self-sufficient. When I started walking more than two minutes a day in what had been my room for so long, it finally hit me that I was bigger than this space. Before I got sick, I never imagined myself leaving Mom's house for good. I knew that she would always serve as my soft place to land. But, with each step, my belief and confidence grew. If I could physically keep one foot in front of the other, on my own—after everything I'd been through—I could begin to take some emotional risks and set out on my own. This room wasn't my final destination. It would not serve as a casket where people would mourn my life and then throw dirt on my purpose. I did not—and would not—take my last breath there. The voices and figures of darkness would not vanish into their abyss with me in tow.

The bed, chair, tiny desk, carpet, and makeshift closet piled together to make one sailboat, gently ebbing me away from all that felt comfortable and familiar, to a gorgeous, vintage apartment that presented adult challenges like paying my own rent and living completely alone for the first time in my forty years.

The morning I left, I wrote Mom a small note in a thank-you card. Over the years, she and I shared a special language in the cards I gave her. She wasn't the type of woman who openly revealed her sentiment through many words. An almost childlike sheepish nature would possess her whenever I paid her a verbal compliment of any kind. She was another Black woman I loved who claimed she didn't need the words. I bypassed what she believed she didn't need to give her what she deserved—my words on paper.

Tears fell faster than I could write. I admired how she offered such a selfless, fierce love that saved my life. As I expressed how thankful I was that she, above anyone else, was the person God designed to care for me, doubt tried to trap me—I had doubts about leaving her. "Maybe I should stay here to help Mom like she helped me? Who do I think I am anyway to just pick up and move the hell out? I could save money by staying. And what will happen to me if I get sick again? Mom will be all the way across town."

Mom's patience, care, will, and belief in God's ability to heal me was what I held onto for nearly two years battling Long COVID. During the moments when my eyes were heaviest and my ears struggled to hear through pain and inflammation, it was her unwavering determination to keep me alive that patched the cracks that death wanted me to fall through.

A cracking did occur. It happened inside of me. I cracked with need. I became greedy for it. I drank from its cup. Feasted on its nourishment. Bathed in the luxury of the magic of expressing a need and it being answered. I became the first Black woman I knew that didn't die from needing someone else.

If anything, needing someone—against my will—provoked my spirit to live. It broke my pride in pieces, making it acceptable to boldly ask for what I wanted and needed, leaving shame behind closed doors I would never open again.

I had needed Mom, as I stood weakly at the bottom of the basement steps, screaming to her words that signaled what I never wanted to reveal: my needs. I not only needed the preacher woman in her to speak to God on my behalf. I also needed her to continue to fight for me. To wave her hands as a sign for death to pull in its wings and back away from our doorstep. To keep the oxygen flowing into breaths that had become harder to take. To defeat the burning stabs at my brain by the vengeful hands of migraines that visited uninvited. To bind the hand of the enemy that had viciously robbed me of sight in my left eye—the eye that doctors repeatedly tried to convince me was just dry.

I needed every morsel of food she prepared, whether I actually ate it or not. The smell alone awakened my dead taste buds, causing me to consider what tiny pleasures might emerge from living for another day.

I needed those cries for God's help that she woefully extended to heaven when she thought I was asleep. Each morning before sunrise, she and her fellow prayer warriors called out the names of church members with loved ones who had either died from the thing that threatened to kill me every second of every day or were suffering at nearby hospitals. Hearing my name meant I was alive—not well or thriving—but alive. That accounted for something. As long as I heard my name commingled in the throes of spiritual tongues and epithets, I knew God was answering Mom, and that he hadn't forgotten me.

I needed her to tell me to "hush" each time I told her I wanted to die. And hush I would. She stopped allowing me to utter the words in her presence. She refused to believe in what I wished for so often.

If I learned anything from Mom, it was that I, too, had the strength to believe in what naturally looked impossible.

For years, I had watched her walk away from the fiery ruins of rejection into the white-hot miracles of acceptance. She had walked into a new church building when bank lenders denied her application. She had walked into pulpits where, before her, only men had been invited. If there ever was a word Mom didn't know, it was the word no. She simply refused to drink from its cup. I had seen seas part because she believed. She didn't know it, but I was taking notes.

Mom had taught me to know when it was time to leave and start anew. She had told stories of deciding to start her own church, buying her first home, becoming one of Baltimore's most respected and recognized bus drivers, burying her youngest son on a Saturday afternoon, then welcoming members to Sunday morning service in the same building. Each of those steps took courage. They weren't bets placed on winning the approval of others. They were chess moves fueled by an awareness of possibility.

For nearly two years, I studied her. Recovering enough to move out on my own—with Long COVID—was a surefire sign that I had passed the test.

Hugging Mom goodbye, I vowed to text her when the movers left my new home. When I settled in my new bed—the first queen-sized one I had ever owned—I sent her a photo of my bedding and curtains. We laughed at it being "my first big girl bed." She told me she was so happy for me. She was so proud of me. I believed her. Even though she was now twenty minutes on the other side of the city, I knew I would always need her. And I would never pretend not to ever again.

Survival Tips

1. Don't be afraid to cry out for help: I still can't believe I actually needed someone, even if that someone was my Mom, a woman I've been so close to for nearly twenty years. Though it was difficult, I'm so thankful that I finally cried out to her for help. I pushed past my Blackness and pride to create the care team I sorely needed.

2. Learn to release shame: Asking for help is easier for some of us than others, but it can be the most freeing step we can take in our healing process. It lifts the burden of shame from us, allowing others to carry us through life's most grueling challenges. And, no matter who we are, we will need to be carried, though we often don't know when or by whom.

3. Expand your definition of caregiver: I can't stress this enough—a caregiver need not be limited to doctors or nurses. No matter how well meaning health care providers may be, they are no match for those who love us already. Yet, we often rely on those we don't know for fear of appearing weak and unbridled to those we do.

4. Expand your definition of asking for help: Asking for help from a caregiver, at first, may not look like asking at all. It may be words pieced together with the only strength you have at the time. More than likely, the people we choose to seek care and compassion from are those who know us a bit anyway, so they may understand if we are unable to fully articulate our needs. Simply expressing need in some form—even through writing—tells our caregivers our stories. It activates our trust in them and, hopefully, ignites empathy within them. Often, we get to choose those who provide us care. I love that.

5. Build a care team: Mom wasn't the only caregiver I sought. But she lit the path for me to consider others. Once I asked her to take care of me, it became easier for me to include my best friend Sequoia, my behavioral therapist Brittany, my biological mother Sandra, and my Aunt Shang onto my care team. Each of them provided essential tools that have aided me over the last two years. In fact, many of these women wondered why I hadn't come to them sooner. From prayers to financial support to mentally unpacking being so ill, each used what makes them so wonderful and accommodating to not only help me, but to engage and challenge me to live. I don't devalue the power of a medical team to support those of us with Long COVID. I just encourage anyone suffering

to never underestimate the power of the people you talk to every single day—including those who may not live with you or share your same physical space. Choosing these women as my support system was and still is better than any medical advice or treatment I've received in two years.

6. Care comes in many forms: Mom cared for and texted me from an upstairs floor, and Sequoia called and texted with me when we couldn't see each other. Care does not have to look like a loved one sitting at your bedside every day. We can ask for help from people next door and people miles away.

7. There is power in needing: We get to choose who cares for us. And that is the most empowering lesson for me. After being denied, rejected, and dejected, I still got to choose. And I'm incredibly thankful I made the right choice. You will, too.

CHAPTER 6

The Obstacle Course

Obtaining a Diagnosis

*Dona Kim Murphey, MD, PhD, Rachel Robles,
and David Putrino*

Dona Kim Murphey,
physician and Long COVID patient

Does a diagnosis matter? I can say that, as a physician, historian of science, community organizer, and especially as a patient who has sought explanations for and relief from my own fluctuating symptoms, it absolutely does. The irony of carrying no official COVID diagnosis despite my abundant work in this space has thrown into very sharp relief what an accurate diagnosis can offer.

As a physician and community organizer, I knew early on that the COVID-19 pandemic would require the creation of robust community resources and support networks. On March 5, 2020, I organized the first community forum on COVID in the Greater Houston area, collaborating with our local NAACP and three television outlets, including Spanish-language media. I invited infectious disease specialists from Baylor College of Medicine and a Chinese American community organizer with a direct pulse on the tragedy unfolding in Wuhan. On March 15, I started a Facebook group interested in prompt, multidisciplinary, data-driven, ethical, and equitable action on this pandemic. It was heavily populated—by design—with health care professionals, elected officials, and community organizers, in addition to members of the public. In the void of publicly accessible scientific reasoning, it ballooned quickly to thirteen thousand members.

By March 16, I was sick. Despite a vast constellation of symptoms well described by early observational studies from Wuhan, China, and Lombardy, Italy, I received no diagnosis. There were no tests at that time. Almost exactly four weeks later, I was contending with a moderate to severe secondary bacterial sinusitis that landed me in two ERs and almost resulted in a hospital admission. Still, I received no diagnosis. While COVID PCR and rapid antigen tests were available by that time, none were run. I am still unclear as to why.

Months into mild, persistent language deficits, intermittent brain fog (see chapter 8), and passive suicidal ideation (see chapter 7), I had the first of what must have been two tiny strokes. As a neurologist and neuroscientist extensively educated on COVID and very aware of the microvascular injury it produces in many organ systems, including the brain, I understood what had likely happened to me. But I had physician colleagues—even friends—express casual skepticism about my claims. I cannot know all the reasons for their doubts, but as an Asian American woman, I was especially attentive to the racialized and gendered stories of erasure from other patients I met through Long COVID education and advocacy. I wonder, also, if an expert-centric medical system played a part in my experience as a patient being invalidated.

I chose not to submit to a full diagnostic workup for stroke at that time; I didn't want to put myself through all of the tests, just to end up without a diagnosis again. I knew microvascular changes wouldn't be visible with any specificity on an MRI and could be missed altogether. The cost of the brain scans was also not trivial, and I knew any resulting recommendations for treatment would have been based on conjecture. Our understanding of COVID was still developing. It wasn't until my second stroke-like episode—over a year after the first—that I agreed to a brain MRI and ended up on secondary stroke prevention (a baby aspirin a day and moderate exercise to control my cholesterol). I was fortunate, by this time, to have among my physician friends a neurologist who had followed the evolving treatments for COVID-related brain injuries and understood the plausibility of my claims.

As a physician, I can state unequivocally the value of diagnosis. Naming a disease is crucial for initiating the proper treatment to reduce symptoms, slow down disease progression, and even save lives. In neurology, a discipline in which we still lack many cures, naming the problem can still empower patients and their families—it can help to validate their suffering, set expectations and prepare them with information about prognoses, connect them to resources and community to navigate the challenges, and introduce them to opportunities to be engaged in clinical research studies, disease registries, or advocacy opportunities. As we still exist in a relative information vacuum with respect to Long COVID, a diagnosis becomes even more critical.

But, diagnosing Long COVID also poses challenges. Diagnosing Long COVID as new, returning, or ongoing symptoms that are present four weeks or more after infection can be problematic, when initial infections are often hard to "prove" due to COVID testing access and reliability issues. What is Long COVID in this context? Can a clinical diagnosis be made without a confirmed test result in the acute phase? Could such a diagnosis consider test positivity (number of positive tests relative to the total number of tests administered) in the community at the time of acute disease to determine probability of infection? Do the providers diagnosing need a patient to describe some constellation of symptoms we can assume was acute COVID? Can a worsening or return of symptoms from well-managed existing chronic illnesses following a COVID infection be diagnosed as Long COVID? For what period of time or in what context should providers and patients continue to attribute symptoms to Long COVID? If we completely ignore the possibility that these nonspecific symptoms might actually have a different origin, we may miss other diagnoses that are dangerous and treatable.

As a scientist, I understand the complexity of diagnosing at a time when there are multiple circulating (non-exclusive) theories about the pathophysiology of Long COVID. The three most common methods of diagnosing Long COVID contain flaws. When attempting to diagnose acute COVID, a molecular diagnosis—typically achieved through a COVID diagnostic PCR test—can detect the presence of viral RNA for up to around 20 days. Similarly, rapid antigen tests can detect the shedding of viral proteins. Both of these tests are most sensitive during a short time window at the beginning of a COVID infection, and for this and other reasons, up to 25 percent of PCR tests and 50 percent of rapid antigen tests result in false negatives. In contrast, an antibody test can confirm the presence of nuclear antibodies, corroborating infection in the months that follow acute COVID (and offering a sense of when the acute infection may have occurred). But not all Long COVID patients produce these antibodies, so these tests cannot be used to rule out a COVID-19 infection. In fact, the absence of antibodies may also be an indicator of Long COVID (see chapter 11).

As a historian of science, I understand the complexity of diagnosis at the system level, where some patients will find it much more difficult to access the appropriate diagnostic workup and care due to economic disadvantage, lack of scientific literacy, insurance denials and health care costs, medical racism, limited English proficiency, health issues that impact one's ability to navigate systems, and profit-centered health care that is driving attrition in medicine, among many other intersecting challenges.

As a community organizer, I understand the complexity of diagnosis at the community level, where mobilizing the people who are marginalized and harmed by a disease can make inroads in diagnosing that disease. Those who are most impacted are highly motivated to confirm the cause of their suffering in order to take more definitive action. We are also most insightful about our illness experiences, which physician researchers have learned to leverage in their evolving understanding of Long COVID and how best to treat it. In the early days of the pandemic, without this partnership, many of us crowd-sourced self-diagnoses by reading other patients' accounts of illness and talking to one another in community forums. Armed with our collective stories, we were better able to demand medical attention and recognition for our illness and popularize a patient-coined name, Long COVID. When people cannot obtain a diagnosis due to structural barriers, organizing to take action can amplify our impact and make the work of seeking diagnoses more sustainable.

In this chapter, we, Dona, Rachel, and David—advocates, patients, and/or providers—will share our specific experiences related to Long COVID diagnosis. We will outline the benefits of obtaining a diagnosis and give you a general framework for doing so, depending on your circumstances.

As this book is meant to provide people with a multitude of disease manifestations with loose guidance on how to live with Long COVID, it would be dishonest to suggest that we will capture all perspectives and concerns. A first step is to acknowledge and confirm that this illness has an expansive definition, which includes people with and without lab test-confirmed COVID-19 infections and a spectrum of symptoms and severity. At its core, Long COVID—which the medical community has renamed with its own esoteric term, *post-acute sequelae SARS-CoV-2 infection* (PASC)—refers to a range of infection-associated illnesses that present as new, returning, or ongoing health problems experienced by people four or more weeks after their initial coronavirus infection. Rarely, similar prolonged symptoms have been reported with SARS-CoV-2 vaccination.

We also must acknowledge the many internal and external ways in which official diagnoses may still elude us. If you do not yet have a diagnosis of Long COVID, there are some important questions to ask yourself before embarking on this journey:

1. Consider your own experiences with Long COVID, not just the physical symptoms of the disease but also the cognitive and psychological aspects. Do you have any fear of diagnoses that may have real consequences for your social or emotional life?

2. Examine the economic aspects of seeking a diagnosis. Does the cost of an exhaustive workup or confirmation of a sometimes significantly disabling and chronic disease that may undermine your economic productivity dissuade you from pursuing a diagnosis?

3. Acknowledge the forces that have shaped your consciousness of your symptoms. Do factors related to your identity and how you have been treated by health care professionals in the past impact your desire to seek care?

There's no right answer to any of these questions, and if they feel daunting to consider, try approaching them in conversation with trusted loved ones or other members of the Long COVID community; peer-to-peer support groups and social media chats can be helpful.

Answers often lie in collective knowledge. Patients and providers alike have been thrust into a new world of post-viral illness, and although many of us were caught off-guard by the emergence of Long COVID, we have been grounded by the patients and clinicians who have faced novel, infection-associated, and complex chronic illnesses before us. In this chapter, we'll take a deep look into the possible causes of Long COVID, keeping in mind the groundwork that has been set up by decades of research and patient experience.

We have also learned that post-viral illnesses cause a spectrum of disability, and asking a house-bound or bed-bound person to use their mental and physical energy on the obstacle course of reaching a diagnosis may not be feasible. If you're living day-to-day just trying to count the little wins and not trigger a relapse, please know that we recognize you. This also goes for those of you who are unable to seek out medical attention due to a lack of time away from work, costs, or other barriers.

No matter what level of ability or privilege you may have (or not have) in seeking out a diagnosis, it's important to find community and advocates to work with. The battle of Long COVID does not stop at its symptoms. For patients, encountering gaslighting, dismissal, and ignorance is often a part of daily life, and the access to social support or a person with the mental energy to help you take on these issues is invaluable. If you or a caregiver has the capacity, we encourage you to soak in as much information about your illness as possible. While there exist many barriers as a result of systemic failings—such as a fifteen-minute limit to doctor's appointments as allowed by insurance—we believe that education is a powerful tool to help bridge gaps. By providing you with the tools to navigate the health care system, we hope to empower you to peel back the layers of your chronic illness to its core, exposing answers to aid you in your healing process.

Why Pursue a Diagnosis?

By putting in the early effort to get answers, you can build a strong foundation to ensure your mental health, physical health, and financial well-being are not being neglected.

MENTAL HEALTH

What happens when an illness that the medical establishment thinks they understand, like COVID, behaves differently in a subset of people, like long-haulers? Unfortunately, often when patients complain of symptoms that are novel or seemingly unusual, they are immediately met with skepticism. Doubts from family, friends, and coworkers seep into their minds, leaving them wondering if their illness is actually "all in their head."

This is where receiving reassurance from a health care provider is key. However, this same skepticism of mysterious-seeming or under-researched illnesses is also pervasive among health care providers. It's not uncommon for a health care provider to make a diagnosis of a somatoform disorder when a patient presents with a physical disorder that has no apparent organic cause. Somatization, which stems from a history of the hysteria diagnosis used to explain (away) illnesses in mostly women, is the belief that emotional distress turns into physical symptoms.

Because somatoform disorders are typically based on symptoms[1] rather than testing criteria, it's convenient for doctors to apply these diagnoses to patients with complex illnesses. Usually, these diagnoses come in the form of "anxiety" or "depression." While these are mental health issues that may accompany chronic illness and can be triggered or worsened by medical gaslighting, they are not the cause of Long COVID. Many Long COVID patients experience this repeatedly, often finding their mental health deteriorating from the emotional toll of being dismissed, as well as from unchecked illness in the central nervous system. They may even give up on trying to find the correct diagnosis—a completely understandable and respectable choice. If you've experienced this, remember that you are not at fault for the failings of systems that deny you care.

For those of you who do continue on your journey to find a diagnosis despite rejection and dismissal, power to you. It is possible—often through recommendations from your chronically ill peers—to find at least one helpful physician who will act in-line with the goals of the medicine practice to promote health and well-being, relieve pain and suffering, and cure disease when possible. After you procure a thoughtful diagnosis, doors open for further care. The right diagnosis can also reassure you that you are not imagining your symptoms or engaging in somatization. Long COVID patients can easily fall through the cracks of the health care system and become invisible. By having an advocate in your health care provider, though, you can ensure that your progress is seen, your voice is heard, and your care is still championed by someone else when you are too sick to do so.

A diagnosis also has the power to inspire hope. When it comes to COVID-19 and Long COVID, there are symptoms that feel urgent and life-threatening, including breathlessness or a rapid heart rate. However, a thoughtful diagnosis like Long COVID, as well as subsequent diagnoses of post-viral conditions such as dysautonomia, ME/CFS, and others, can help to assure you that (1) there may be no cause for immediate concern and (2) there are ways to manage those frightening symptoms. For issues not under the realm of a health care provider's guidance, such as personal experiences and feelings, finding community, coping strategies, or firsthand information about treatments, support groups can provide an invaluable resource for upholding your mental health.

On that note, we recognize it seems counterintuitive to suggest that the very thing that may be worsening your mental health struggles, the health care system, will help support your mental health (see chapter 7). For many, such as women, people of color, and people in larger bodies, we acknowledge that this is a hurdle that may be too high to get past. It is our hope that by arming you with the best tools possible, you can break past these barriers. Once you have access to a trusted provider, you gain the power to receive more specialized tests that can lead to a diagnosis for Long COVID or its comorbidities.

Once your condition is named and treated, you might find that your mental health improves as a result. Because mental health challenges are a byproduct of Long COVID—not the cause—optimal mental health can only be achieved when emotional well-being practices are done in tandem with addressing the root illness.

PHYSICAL HEALTH

Addressing the root illness is a tall order for Long COVID. Since there is no magic cure-all, each person must devise their own plan based on their short- and long-term goals for recovery—which can only happen once the condition is named. Then, the patient chooses their own adventure based on what will impact their physical health most. When dealing with this crossroads in something as complex as Long COVID, you and your health care providers may be confronted with a multitude of questions.

In the short-term, you might not be looking for a cure, but instead a way to stabilize your health to be able to live a functional life. If this is the case, you'll need to find answers to the following questions:

1. **Are there any treatment options for specific symptoms preventing me from sleeping, eating, being mobile, etc.?** You can ask this of a physician during an appointment when they ask about your goals for the visit. It may be helpful to further define what types of treatment you're comfortable with, as some people favor rehabilitation or another type of intervention over medication.

2. **What accommodations can be made at work, home, and elsewhere so I can perform daily functions while managing my symptoms?** Utilizing resources like the Job Accommodation Network[2] or support groups can be helpful to provide suggestions. You can learn more about options for receiving disability benefits in chapter 4.

As you proceed on your journey to make your daily life manageable, you may want to start looking for longer-term solutions. (Note: This is not always the case. Many chronically ill people don't have enough physical, mental, or emotional energy to get to this point, so this is where caregivers and other loved ones may step in if desired.) Here, you may need to find answers to the following questions:

1. **Are there any treatment options for addressing the root cause of my illness?** You can ask this question when your health care provider asks about your goals for the visit, but note that this will likely open up a larger conversation. When the pathogenesis of an illness has yet to be defined, there are no treatments that are guaranteed to cure the disease. However, there are treatments that have worked for other people with infection-associated illnesses or that have shown some effectiveness for Long COVID patients in clinical trials, such as hyperbaric oxygen therapy,[3] vagus nerve stimulation,[4] and stem cell therapy,[5] which may be explored if a physician recommends it. You can also bring research papers on these therapies to your provider to start such a conversation (for more on how to do this, see chapter 11). This may prompt a discussion about how you can be involved as a subject in ongoing research, since it can be tiring to continually be waiting for insights to come out of clinical trials.

2. **Are there any research opportunities to get access to better testing or treatment for my diagnosis?** Research is often conducted upon rigid inclusion criteria. While Long COVID advocates recommend positive tests not be included in criteria for the accuracy and accessibility issues mentioned in the first part of this chapter (for more on this, see page 116), there are still many studies in which that is the case. Life-changing rehabilitation, medications, and testing are among the modalities being researched, and any evidence you can provide to prove your Long COVID case is crucial for accessing those options.

3. **How can I build better health for myself?** This question can be brought to your trusted health care provider, as well as any holistic medicine provider, such as a nutritionist, acupuncturist, or integrative/functional medicine specialist. Functional medicine testing can be especially helpful in identifying dysfunctions in the body that standard diagnostics miss, such as gut dysbiosis (an imbalance of bacteria in your gut), mitochondrial dysfunction (a disruption in the ability of the body's cells to produce energy), and oxidative stress (changes to the chemical balance of cells that can cause damage). Together, these providers can help optimize your nutrition, sleep hygiene, and other aspects of your life to help you build a foundation for better wellness.

After receiving a diagnosis, you can use these questions to identify all of your options. You may start taking a daily inhaler to manage your asthma, embark on a diet and lifestyle change to build a foundation for better health, or enroll in a clinical trial for the newest pharmaceutical innovation. With a diagnosis, you have the power to take control of your physical health.

FINANCIAL WELL-BEING

A diagnosis can also help ease the burden of financial responsibility. As many of us know, being sick is not cheap. When an illness starts to transition from acute to chronic, the path to relief becomes daunting as each appointment and supplement results in a new bill or charge to your credit card.

There are many types of financial and legal support that can help you navigate the financial burden of chronic illness and disability—but many require a diagnosis. If you are unable to keep or pursue a job, it is imperative that you document all diagnoses from a doctor to help make the case for any disability income and benefits that you applied for. For more information, please refer to chapter 4.

If you have health insurance, receiving a diagnosis is essential for insurance to pay for specific testing, treatments, or visits with specialists. Tests that go beyond basic blood work and imaging are often met with opposition by insurance companies, who sometimes argue that such tests are experimental. In these cases, utilizing diagnostic codes can be helpful. The *International Classification of Diseases* (ICD) is a tool that assigns codes for diseases, symptoms, abnormal findings, and other circumstances. When navigating ICD, insurance companies expect consistency between a diagnosis and the treatment rendered for it. For example, if a person is prescribed a migraine medication but the provider doesn't submit the correct diagnosis code, the insurance company can deny the claim.

In October 2021, Long COVID received an ICD-10 code, currently U09.9, which can be utilized by physicians to bill insurance companies for payment of appointments, testing, services rendered, and, one day, treatments. But because there are no approved treatments for Long COVID, insurance companies may refuse to pay for any treatments that are filed solely under that diagnosis code. In this case, your provider should list multiple codes for all of your relevant symptoms; you can advocate for this during or after an appointment. For example, if you're dealing with worsened eczema as a result of Long COVID, you may want to make sure you receive a diagnosis for eczema, and that your provider utilizes the appropriate ICD-10 codes to make a case for insurance to cover any eczema-related treatments.

If you're seeking services that are subjective when it comes to insurance coverage, such as an appointment with a nutritionist, you may want to call your insurance company beforehand to understand in what circumstances these services will be covered. Oftentimes, insurance will only cover these appointments if certain diagnostic codes are used, which justify a medical need for the appointment. These codes can be found anywhere you can access the provider's notes from your appointment, whether that be via a patient portal, a summary of your visit that arrives by mail, or a superbill—a detailed invoice outlining the services received, which you can submit to your insurance if a provider doesn't correspond with insurance companies directly.

Insurance company approval can be subjective, and they can deny your payments even if the correct diagnostic codes are used. In these circumstances, you can make an appeal to your insurance company to further explain how the diagnostic codes used justify the use and coverage of certain tests or treatments.

Rachel Robles,
Long COVID patient and advocate

IT WAS MID-MARCH of 2020. The world around me was shutting down as the coronavirus pandemic took hold in New York City. Just like every other March, during the peak of allergy season, my asthma was flaring up. I used my inhaler if I needed to but otherwise waited for the symptoms to run their course. As the days passed by, though, my asthma was somehow worsening. Despite multiple trips to urgent care, a prescription for Montelukast, and a course of steroids, my lungs began to feel like they were on fire.

A few days later, I awoke to a low-grade fever, a headache, a backache, nausea, and fatigue. To my surprise, I had absolutely no respiratory symptoms—I was breathing more clearly than I had in two weeks. Yet, my body no longer felt in my control. I felt like a passenger in a vehicle driven erratically in circles by a pathogen I could not yet name. That day, I realized I was no longer dealing with an average case of seasonal asthma. My symptoms, while wildly unpredictable, presented like COVID, so I decided to cuddle up on the couch and rest. Based on the media's portrayal of the illness at the time, I assumed it would be about a week before I could get back to normal life. After all, I was young and in great physical shape, having just completed my first half marathon less than a year prior. *Surely*, I thought, *people like me don't get extremely sick from COVID-19.*

Testing wasn't widely available, and people without serious preexisting conditions were being told to stay at home and treat themselves, in order to not overwhelm hospitals and clinics. So, I stayed home. That first week came and went, and my illness remained mild. But the second week tore apart my perceived level of health. My difficulty breathing became debilitating. My inhaler—typically a lifeline to anyone with asthma—stopped producing any results at the moments I needed it most. Because I lived by myself, and the hospitals closest to me were overburdened, I wasn't confident that help would get to me fast enough if I needed it, a shocking and terrifying realization. After some tears, wheezing, and panic on my worst night of symptoms, my breathing slowly stabilized, allowing me to see another day in the comfort of my own home. Through virtual urgent care and pulmonology appointments, I received reassurance and a care plan from doctors. My urgent care telehealth doctors, who acknowledged that the health care system was on the verge of collapsing, diagnosed me with a presumed COVID-19 infection and prescribed medications aimed at minimizing inflammation in my lungs and body. They told me I'd been "spared from the worst of it" and urged me to sit at home and wait it out.

Since then, over two years have passed. I am still waiting it out.

In March 2020, with a pandemic unfolding around me, I scoured the internet for any information on how to recover from a COVID-19 infection. The days passed, and my difficulty breathing, fatigue, headaches, low-grade fevers, body aches, and brain fog continued. Virtual urgent care providers continued to reassure me that my illness would resolve soon and prescribed more medications to manage my symptoms and quell any secondary infections.

After about two months, I decided to search for specialists with expertise in infectious diseases. In a stark contrast to the validation I'd gotten from the urgent care telehealth providers, I received diagnosis after diagnosis of anxiety from these specialists, because I didn't have a positive COVID-19 diagnostic test. At the beginning of my illness, I was given a clinical diagnosis of COVID-19, despite not having access to testing. Now, the very symptoms that had informed that diagnosis were weaponized against me. On one visit to an infectious disease specialist, I was told, "COVID-19 doesn't last for ninety days. You either get over it, or you die."

Desperate and defeated, with few options for my recovery, I grew weary. It was then that I read about a patient-led support group for COVID-19 patients in *The New York Times*. In the group, themes of dismissal and outrage popped up again and again. Other patients described having to fend for themselves because they too weren't able to receive a positive test. My experience had not been an outlier, but rather part of a long-standing tradition of health care providers ignoring post-viral illnesses. Standard blood tests and imaging are often not granular enough to detect abnormalities like the ones experts believe exist in Long COVID patients—pathogens hiding in tissues, microvascular damage, and mitochondrial dysfunction, to name a few—and without a curious provider, the investigation stops there. Patients are told "everything's normal," and given medications to suppress their symptoms.

Through this online community of patients, I became empowered to be my own advocate. At their recommendation, I sought out any provider who would believe me and was curious to learn more, and hired them. I researched post-viral conditions such as ME/CFS and dysautonomia and found providers who were literate in those conditions. While it may seem excessive to seek out so many specialists, this practice, when possible, can be essential for people with mysterious-seeming illnesses and symptoms. It certainly was for me.

As I connected with more providers and further pursued relief and—I hoped—some form of recovery, I had to make some difficult choices. While medications that help suppress symptoms can be important for reducing pain and allowing patients to function, these fixes sometimes come with side effects and often don't address a symptom's underlying cause. I decided early on that I only wanted medication if it was treating a possible cause—a condition upstream that had a hand in causing the cascading effect of Long COVID. For example, some Long COVID symptoms are partially a result of reactivated viruses; I decided I would consider pursuing treatments that targeted this cause. I went to many doctor appointments, often leaving with prescriptions for medications treating migraines, nausea, and eczema, but no closer to answers.

Despite the heartache and trauma associated with telling an illness origin story over and over again only to be dismissed, I continued on my journey for better medical attention. About three months into my illness, I went to a cardiologist, and left with a feeling of vindication and victory after receiving my first post-viral diagnosis: postural orthostatic tachycardia syndrome (POTS).

While the cause of post-viral POTS is being researched and debated, its diagnosis is still critical. Its hallmark symptoms, such as rapid heart rate, dizziness upon standing, nausea, and brain fog, are often falsely attributed to anxiety, which can leave the patient untreated or mistreated. Equipped with new knowledge from my specialist, I started implementing practices in my life to manage the condition (and the symptoms associated with it). I took beta-blockers and salt capsules, increased my water intake, and worked from a supine position. I learned what my biggest dysautonomia triggers were—my menstrual cycle, warm weather, blood draws, anesthesia, and standing for long periods of time—and found ways to mitigate symptoms when confronted with these triggers. By obtaining that diagnosis and managing my post-viral illness, I've been able to live my life with minimal dysautonomia-related symptoms. To those unfamiliar with the illness, this may seem like a small victory, but for me, it was a giant step toward relief and recovery.

I then shifted my focus to investigate my other ailments. While standard blood work was consistently coming up clean, test results from my infectious disease specialist, who also has expertise in ME/CFS, showed a drastically different picture. My immune function had been compromised by my COVID-19 infection, showing low humoral response, heightened T-cell response, and low-grade systemic inflammation. COVID-19 had reactivated other viruses in my body, which were previously kept in check by my immune system. These viruses, specifically Epstein-Barr virus and human herpesvirus 6 (HHV-6), were thought to be driving some of my Long COVID symptoms. I considered the diagnoses of these viruses to be a possible root cause and began an antiviral treatment to target the infections. Within a few days, I noticed that my ribs no longer felt confined. For the first time in nine months, I was able to take a full, deep breath.

At this point, it was clear there were multiple mechanisms at play in my post-viral illness. The depth of my Long COVID seemed endless, and I wondered what other answers I could uncover. Continuing the exploration upstream, I searched for more answers to the dysfunctions that my chronic symptoms alluded to.

Months went by as I grappled with the reality of living my daily life with disabilities. I spent my weekdays logging onto my laptop for my job, which entailed answering emails, running meetings, and coding, only to be met with extreme head pressure, tinnitus, low-grade fevers, and migraines. I was forced to pace my screen time, as any amount over my threshold (the amount I could tolerate without experiencing worsened symptoms, which happened to be about forty-five minutes of engaging work or two hours of passive work) would derail me by hours or days. As I became more familiar with the concept of post-exertional symptom exacerbation (also known as post-exertional malaise, or PEM) from my support group, I observed my symptom relapses closely. PEM generally occurs after physical, emotional, or cognitive activities (or all three); my relapses were triggered primarily by screen usage. This realization prompted me to do some research and field the expertise of my care team and fellow patients. They found that my screen sensitivity, along with other symptoms I experienced daily, aligned heavily with post-concussion syndrome (PCS).

Whether it's through damage to nerves, damage from blood clots, or other currently speculated causes, COVID-19 has been shown to threaten the brain.[6] Despite having a clean MRI three months into my illness, I continually experienced symptoms of brain fog that caused difficulties reading text, understanding conversations, focusing, and retaining and recalling short-term memories. Several times, as I rode the subway to doctor appointments, I forgot where I was and where the train was heading.

Motivated by my suspicions around PCS causing a cascade of symptoms, I found a concussion clinic familiar with the impact of viruses on brains, as well as post-viral conditions such as dysautonomia. At the clinic, I received a functional MRI (fMRI) to measure the blood flow inside my brain. The results, which showed that certain parts of my brain were hyperactive while others were hypoactive, found dysfunction in the cerebral cortex, a part of the brain that plays a key role in attention, perception, awareness, thought, memory, language, and consciousness.

I met three out of the possible five biomarkers for brain injury, indicating that my neural activation patterns, which should have been working throughout the day to keep my attention focused and thoughts succinct, were less than ideal. I imagined signals in my brain taking a long, winding detour just to get me to remember the word for *refrigerator* or *compromise*. These pathways in my brain were so inefficient, which meant that my neural systems required a greater amount of energy and resources to function. This resulted in symptoms like migraines, fatigue, and sensitivity to sounds.

To remedy the symptoms of brain injury, they put me through an intensive and varied treatment plan. For a week, I engaged in physical exercise, meditation, cognitive tests, breathing exercises, balancing activities, and massages. The therapists taught me how to utilize interval training and breathing exercises simultaneously to raise and then lower my heart rate, which strengthened my nervous system in the process. Leading up to the visit at the clinic, I had been able to go on walks without any symptom exacerbation or significant increase in heart rate, so they allowed me to challenge myself with a thirty- to forty-five-second run. (For people dealing with significant PEM after physical activity like short walks, this treatment would likely be less appropriate.)

The goal of the exercise is to do an action that tests the boundaries for *you*, without going over your personal energy envelope, and then doing calming, structured breathing exercises. Some people choose a slow walk on the treadmill. Others do supine exercises. In cognitive therapy—not to be confused with cognitive behavioral therapy (CBT), which is sometimes inaccurately prescribed as a cure for post-viral illnesses—the specialists gave me specific cognitive challenges to do, such as naming a country for every letter of the alphabet while listening to background noises, to condition my brain to be less sensitive to distractions. By the end of the week, my fMRI showed drastic improvements in the blood flow within my brain, and in the following months, I was able to reap the benefits of my hard work. Because I was able to identify and treat my brain injury, I walked away from the clinic with more stable energy, the ability to withstand loud noises, and better short-term memory and concentration, among other improvements.

Even though my self-advocacy was, and remains, soaked in blood, sweat, and tears, every thoughtful diagnosis I've received since becoming ill with COVID-19 has helped ease the pain of my suffering. With the help of my COVID-literate doctors, many of whom see the value in systemic approaches, I've been able to diagnose some of the damage done by the virus, co-infections that have weakened my body, and an immune system that was put into overdrive. Like many post-viral patients, I am still trekking on the path to full recovery, taking many different avenues in the hopes of someday finding an express lane to full health.

In the meantime, I've found relief by continuing my search for the root causes of my illness while simultaneously working on building my health from the ground up. I've seen an increasing number of health care providers who believe in treating the whole body—not just the parts—which has propelled me forward in my journey. This functional and integrative approach emphasizes the use of testing to understand the body's ecosystem as well as evidence-based and data-driven approaches. With this framework, I've pursued providers and clinical trials and have participated in Long COVID-related research to understand more about my illness and have gained access to testing that exposes what my body needs on a cellular level. This has opened the doors for me to address possible root causes of illness, like mitochondrial dysfunction or viral persistence.

To build my health, acupuncture, craniosacral therapy, diaphragmatic breathing exercises, and EMDR have all been staple therapies for me to manage my chronic symptoms and the anxiety, depression, and PTSD that come alongside a chronic illness. I try to optimize my sleep hygiene, nutritional intake, and mental health practices to limit symptoms and soothe my nervous system. I eat a low-histamine diet, engage in a nightly, screen-free sleep routine for thirty minutes, and pursue my passions: singing a cappella and doing gymnastics. I want to acknowledge that such lifestyle interventions can be difficult or impossible to implement, and even in the best circumstances, are only added gradually over time! With my unpredictable symptoms and limited time, incorporating these changes is a constant task. While maintaining these practices has been key to gradually building my health, I have found that a meaningful diagnosis has been just as important.

David Putrino,
Associate Professor, Department of Rehabilitation and Human Performance, Icahn School of Medicine at Mount Sinai, New York City

IN THE FIRST FEW WEEKS of March 2020, New York City was in the midst of the first wave of SARS-CoV-2 infection. My team at the Abilities Research Center (often called the "ARC") at Mount Sinai was busy preparing for incoming patients. We set up emergency triage tents, were deployed into the hospital in all sorts of roles that ranged from treating critically ill patients to delivering hot meals, snacks, and water to exhausted essential workers, and created "Recharge Rooms" for staff to process the trauma they were experiencing across the hospital system. However, we knew that there was a critical need that was still unmet: After people came to our emergency departments with COVID symptoms and were told that they were "not sick enough" to be admitted to the hospital, what was next?

In non-pandemic times, the role of the ARC is to rapidly develop new technologies to help people living with neurological conditions. We are trained to develop technology in a hurry. In the past, the ARC had created a remote patient monitoring technology called Precision Recovery, an app that kept track of stroke survivors once they had left the hospital and ensured that they were maintaining safe blood pressures and staying well. We quickly saw the potential to use the same platform (with a few key changes) to keep COVID patients safe, so on March 15, the ARC started monitoring COVID patients in their homes.

The referrals came in thick and fast, and within a few short weeks our team was monitoring hundreds of acutely ill people with COVID. Each day, we had a huddle in which we'd discuss tricky situations—talking through particularly sick patients or unusual COVID symptoms that were emerging. By early May, it was evident that some of our patients undergoing monitoring were staying in the monitoring app longer than expected. Usually, people with acute COVID dropped off the app within three to four weeks of monitoring, without further issues. However, this wasn't the case for 10 to 15 percent of Precision Recovery users. Not only did they continue monitoring their symptoms daily, but they also started to report an entirely new cluster of symptoms: extreme fatigue, cognitive difficulties, body pains, post-exertional symptom exacerbation, persistent shortness of breath, and many other issues that we now know are hallmarks of Long COVID. We began to realize that the Precision Recovery program couldn't help these people, and we also didn't have a plan for how to treat them.

The Diagnostic Framework

As the number of patients struggling to recover from acute COVID cases kept increasing, my team knew that we were facing something novel and complex.

In response, we began the process of building a new task force to tackle this issue. One of the major benefits of my job, even prior to the pandemic, is that I have the privilege of working with an incredibly diverse team. On any given day, members of my group might engage with elite athletes, kids or adults with complex, multisystem conditions, people living with severe paralysis, and many other diverse populations. As a result, it's necessary for members of my team to have access to a world-class and interdisciplinary group of professionals.

The task force we initially created to address the new influx of patients consisted of two clinicians with Long COVID, two psychiatrists, a cardiologist, a strength and conditioning coach, two physical therapists (one with pulmonary and one with neurology specialties), a registered dietician, and two neuroscientists. The term *Long COVID* didn't yet exist, so we came up with our own name for the condition. In collaboration with a collective of physicians with Long COVID in the United Kingdom, led by a wonderful physician named Clare Rayner (who had developed Long COVID after contracting COVID while working on the front lines of the pandemic with the UK's National Health Service), we arrived at the name *Post-Acute COVID-19 Syndrome* or PACS.

The next step was to develop a framework for care. Whether you're a person trying to manage an unknown condition that you're living with or a clinician trying to treat it, there are usually two angles from which you can work the problem:

1. Person-facing: What are the main symptoms that are affecting daily function? How can you best address those symptoms to provide short-term relief?

2. Physiology-facing: What is the pathophysiology (underlying cause) of the condition? What is the body doing to produce the symptoms that the patient is experiencing?

Our team at Mount Sinai knew we had limited time and resources; the people using our app needed assistance immediately, and their numbers were growing. So, our first approach was person-facing: to catalog symptoms. We sent questionnaires to thousands of people who were reporting post-acute symptoms and analyzed the data to develop an understanding about what they were dealing with. The first insight that emerged was that many people with Long COVID were reporting symptoms consistent with a condition called dysautonomia.

DYSAUTONOMIA

Dysautonomia is an umbrella term for many different symptoms that can be explained by dysfunction of the autonomic nervous system, the part of the human nervous system that does a lot of things in the background "autonomously" (i.e., without requiring conscious effort) to keep our body functioning.

For instance, when we decide to move our body from sitting to standing, we make a conscious choice to move, but in the background our autonomic nervous system works as our silent copilot. It alters our blood pressure so that our brain is getting the same amount of blood when we're standing as it was when we were sitting, and it typically does this by *very slightly* dialing up our heart rate. In people with postural orthostatic tachycardia syndrome (POTS), a type of dysautonomia, the delicate heart rate "dial" that ensures that their blood pressure is appropriate for standing is damaged. Instead, when they stand up, their heart rate and blood pressure become erratic and they can experience dizziness, fuzzy vision, feeling like they're going to faint, and more—all brought about by something as simple as changing positions.

If these symptoms sound familiar to you, you're not alone: More than 80 percent of people with Long COVID report signs and symptoms that are consistent with dysautonomia. Furthermore, there is strong evidence that certain types of rehabilitation and lifestyle changes that focus on autonomic nervous system regulation can ease (not cure) Long COVID symptoms. However, we must never lose sight of the fact that while dysautonomia is an explanation of sorts, it doesn't explain all of the Long COVID symptoms that we are seeing, and it certainly does not tell us why the virus has caused the autonomic nervous system to malfunction. For this, we need physiology-facing research.

Physiology-Facing Research

As we search for a mechanism to explain why people are experiencing such intense and debilitating Long COVID symptoms, it's important to acknowledge that the information presented here may change as we learn more. Currently, there are three leading theories on what may be causing Long COVID symptoms, and they are as follows:

I. **Autoimmunity:** The physiological response brought about by the acute COVID-19 infection triggers a reaction in which the body's immune system is confused and begins to attack itself.

2. **Chronic inflammation:** In many, acute COVID-19 produces an extreme inflammatory response (sometimes called a cytokine storm), and in some people, the inflammation doesn't easily resolve, which produces long-term symptoms.

3. **Viral persistence:** The COVID-19 virus doesn't fully clear the body and produces immune reactions and damage all over the body.

This knowledge is still evolving. It's possible that none of these theories are correct, or that all three pathological processes are occurring simultaneously. It's also possible that some cases of Long COVID are a result of one of these processes and other cases of Long COVID result from others. Additionally, many of us who are reading the emerging Long COVID literature or who have lived experience will come across multiple other diagnoses, such as mast cell activation syndrome (MCAS), a condition where people experience prolonged symptoms that are consistent with a severe allergic reaction; vagus nerve dysfunction, dysautonomia caused by damage to the vagus nerve, a peripheral nerve that manages many of our autonomic functions; POTS; endothelial dysfunction, impaired functioning of blood vessels; and many others.

But there is good science to suggest that the three leading theories might be the underlying cause of many of these diagnoses. For the sake of keeping this chapter accessible, we're not going to discuss every potential diagnosis that people with Long COVID may be facing right now. The list is too long, and knowledge gaps still exist, but it is our hope that we might provide some level of insight into how the physiology of a person with Long COVID can produce such diverse, debilitating symptoms that affect multiple organ systems and body parts.

As we begin to explore the underlying causes of Long COVID, it's also important for us to acknowledge and learn from the decades of existing literature investigating the physiology underlying infection-associated illness and autoimmunity. There is much that we can learn from communities that have been living with and studying ME/CFS, Lyme disease, Epstein-Barr virus, dysautonomia, and a multitude of autoimmune conditions for decades. The team at the

Abilities Research Center has collaborated with a number of world-leading physicians and scientists in these fields, and together we are working rapidly with
the Long COVID community to investigate some of these avenues.

AUTOIMMUNITY AND CHRONIC INFLAMMATION

Shortly after the Mount Sinai team published a Long COVID paper in August of
2020, Dr. Akiko Iwasaki from Yale University reached out to collaborate. Akiko is a legendary immunologist who has had a distinguished career studying
how viruses can have long-term effects on the immune system (you can read
more about her work, in her own words, in this book's afterword). Together
with Akiko's team, Mount Sinai's team is conducting research that is confirming
what many other immunology research teams are also reporting: The majority
of Long COVID patients, in comparison to healthy controls and individuals who
have fully recovered from COVID, have abnormally high levels of inflammatory
cytokines (cells that our bodies produce during an inflammatory response) and
autoantibodies (a substance our bodies produce that can attack the body's own
tissues).

The challenge researchers face thus far with these discoveries is that there are
currently no consistent patterns in the way that the bodies of people with Long
COVID are producing inflammatory cytokines and autoantibodies. One person
with Long COVID will show high levels of autoantibody and cytokine production
that is consistent with damage to the central nervous system, while others may
show autoantibodies and cytokines that interact with the gastrointestinal tract.
Although this inconsistency is troubling, focusing on the symptoms that people
with Long COVID are experiencing may hold the key. For instance, a recent
collaboration between teams led by Dr. Michelle Monje, Akiko, and me showed
that people with Long COVID who self-report cognitive symptoms tended to
have higher levels of a specific cytokine called CCL11 compared to people with
Long COVID who do not report cognitive symptoms.

As we move toward a better understanding of abnormal cytokine and autoantibody production in people with Long COVID, it's important to note that
these findings support a more collaborative approach between people with
Long COVID and health care providers. If physicians can use the most severe
symptoms being reported by people with Long COVID to guide the specific

autoantibody and cytokine testing that is performed, we may find ourselves in a situation where fewer people with Long COVID are given the news that, despite experiencing severe and debilitating symptoms, they are "testing normal."

VIRAL PERSISTENCE

From Epstein-Barr to Zika virus, there's a rich body of literature to suggest that, in many cases of viral infection, a virus can continue to live in different tissues of the human body for years after the initial acute infection. This is the concept of viral persistence. My team has had the privilege of exploring this possibility with Dr. Amy Proal, a microbiologist from the PolyBio Research Foundation, and Dr. Saurabh Mehandru, a gastroenterologist from Mount Sinai. Saurabh has published remarkable work showing that people with Long COVID who have persistent gastrointestinal symptoms showed evidence of having living virus in their gastrointestinal tracts.

Indeed, many researchers have discovered that people with Long COVID show evidence of viral persistence in their tissues but, unfortunately, so do people who have fully recovered from COVID. As a result, the role that persistent virus plays on symptom presentation remains unclear. A new collaboration between the Mount Sinai team, Saurabh, and Amy will focus on using more advanced genetic techniques not just to identify the presence of viral persistence, but also to understand whether the persistent virus is *interacting* with the tissue where it's found. It is our hope that this will lead to a better understanding of how the presence of persistent virus is associated with the symptoms of Long COVID.

MICROCLOTS

A new and remarkable finding in the field of Long COVID has been made recently by Dr. Resia Pretorius, a biologist at Stellenbosch University in South Africa. In recent publications, Resia's team has shown that people with Long COVID consistently show evidence of microthrombi (small clots) in their bloodstream. These clots aren't large enough to block major blood vessels or cause life-threatening events, but they are large enough to affect the function of multiple organs in a more insidious way.

My team, along with a community of people with Long COVID led by Dr. Asad Kahn, a UK-based physician with Long COVID, Resia's team, and an international team of many other phenomenal researchers (affectionately referred to online as "#TeamCLOTS") have shown that the severity of microthrombi presentation can correlate strongly with the objective severity of Long COVID symptoms.

Furthermore, there is early pilot research that suggests that a therapeutic technique called heparin-induced extracorporeal LDL precipitation (HELP-apheresis), which has been pioneered for people with Long COVID by Dr. Beate Jaeger in Germany, can reduce the presentation of microclots in the blood of people with Long COVID and has been associated with an improvement in their symptoms. Although this is a slight oversimplification, HELP-apheresis can be thought of as a technique that passes a person's blood through a filter that specifically removes microclots and inflammatory molecules. Apheresis is not a technique to be taken lightly, it's rather invasive and carries certain risks, but for many years it has been used safely to treat other systemic conditions such as certain cancers, autoimmune conditions, and cholesterol disorders.

Although this research is still in its very early stages at the time of this writing, the early results for people with Long COVID have been promising. One aspect to note, however, is that work from the #TeamCLOTS collective has also shown that microclot formation continues in people with Long COVID within twenty-four hours of undergoing apheresis. This indicates that microclots are a *symptom* of Long COVID, not the underlying cause. Our next step is to figure out why and how people with Long COVID are producing microclots in their blood.

If there's any one consistent truth in the field of biomedical research, it's that for every question we answer, we encounter several more that need to be answered. This pattern will continue until we have a unified theory for the complex and puzzling condition known as Long COVID. We are grateful for the hard work of the exceptional scientists and clinicians that we've encountered on this journey, as well as the incredible force of the patient-led research that has helped us reach this point. It is our hope that, as we continue collaborating and searching for answers, we do not lose this crucial and open dialogue between researchers, physicians, and the Long COVID community.

How to Obtain an Accurate Diagnosis

When navigating the world of Long COVID, one of the most beneficial things a patient can do is to find a trusted health care provider who is kind, knowledgeable, and curious. While it's easier to be a patient when you have the trust of your physicians, it's still possible to advocate for yourself in the opposite circumstance. If you ever find yourself in a medical setting where you are being gaslit, here are some helpful questions you can ask that may prompt the physician to reexamine their diagnosis:

1. "What is your differential diagnosis for my condition?" A differential diagnosis is a method of analysis of a patient's history and physical examination to arrive at the correct diagnosis. For any symptom, such as a chronic cough, there may be many differential diagnoses that need to be ruled out to arrive at the correct diagnosis.

2. "What is the evidence for and against that differential?"

3. "How have you ruled these differential diagnoses out?"

4. "Could you please document that?"

By asking for a differential diagnosis, you are asking the provider to logically outline their thought process and be thorough in ruling out possible causes. Hopefully, this encourages more providers to rethink their diagnoses and embark on a thorough investigation.

You can also arm yourself with information about specific tests to ask a physician to order, from common tests that check on the health of major organs while fighting a pathogen to more abstract tests if the former all come up clean. When dealing with illnesses that do not have an understood pathophysiology, nobody has a comprehensive guide. Physicians have their toolboxes but may not know how to go beyond their existing knowledge, especially when a patient's exams appear normal. It is at this point that we can turn to research and collective patient experience for guidance.

When you're on a quest to obtain a diagnosis, outlining your goals is crucial. If you've been sick for two years and suspect that you might have been initially infected with COVID-19, you may have a goal to determine if you have Long COVID or another post-viral or bacterial illness. On the other hand, if you're a patient with Long COVID who hasn't fully recovered and is wondering why and what you can do to address your symptoms, you may be searching for a diagnosis that points to a root cause of your Long COVID symptoms. Both circumstances are equally valid.

To help you in your search for a Long COVID diagnosis, we offer a framework for retrieving an initial COVID-19 diagnosis and then guidance thereafter if symptoms persist.

INITIAL COVID OR LONG COVID DIAGNOSIS

During acute infection (if COVID-19 symptoms are present)

1. Take a rapid antigen and/or PCR test to confirm the presence of a COVID infection.

- If positive, that test result can validate Long COVID diagnosis should symptoms persist.

- If negative, you can retest every few days while symptomatic. If it remains negative, but you still suspect it is COVID, you may want to go to a doctor to get a clinical diagnosis on the record. Having a documented COVID-19 infection will make it easier to diagnose Long COVID should symptoms persist.

2. Request additional tests: complete blood count, basic metabolic panel, liver function tests, thyroid function tests for constitutional symptoms, chest X-ray for respiratory symptoms.

Around 120 days after symptoms of COVID-19 arise

1. Nuclear antibody testing can confirm natural infection.

- If positive, that test result can validate a Long COVID diagnosis should symptoms persist or appear after a few months.

- If negative, it may be because of the test's accuracy or lack of seroconversion (an inability to create antibodies) within the patient.

2. Request additional tests: complete blood count, basic metabolic panel, liver function tests, thyroid function tests for constitutional symptoms, chest X-ray for respiratory symptoms.

These tests are helpful in assessing your initial infection and immune response, but they don't do much to address the cascading effect of Long COVID should it occur. Because of this, we offer another framework to dig deeper into underlying causes of the illness. It's important to note that, because the pathogenesis of this illness has not yet been defined, there is no clear-cut or one-size-fits-all approach. If you want to get to the root of your illness, you may have to do some further investigation specific to your case.

LONG COVID THEORY APPROACH

1. Autoimmunity: Some autoantibody panels are widely available, while others are hard to come by. If the basic autoimmunity screenings, such as antinuclear antibodies (ANA) and tests for autoimmune diseases, come back negative and your health care providers suspect that autoimmunity is a cause of your illness, it may be beneficial to seek out an experienced rheumatologist or immunologist who can run a more nuanced analysis. You can also seek out clinical trials where more specialized autoantibody and immune function tests are being conducted.

2. Chronic inflammation: There are many widely available tests that check for systemic inflammation, such as C-reactive protein (CRP) and erythrocyte sedimentation rate (ESR). If those tests come up clean, it may even be worth it to check high-sensitivity C-reactive protein (hs-CRP), which can find lower levels of C-reactive protein. Cytokine panels are similar to autoantibody panels in that some are widely available, while others are hard to come by. Cytokine Panel 13 can be easily ordered and will identify elevated levels of specific cytokines, which modulate the inflammatory response.

3. Viral persistence: As mentioned on page 136, work is currently being done in research settings through the testing of tissue samples to check for the existence of viral particles. This means that the best bet for finding these tests is by enrolling in clinical trials. It's also possible to find the researchers looking into these questions who have clinical practices; they may have the tools to run these tests outside of a research setting.

4. Other theories:
   - Gut microbiome is out of whack (dysbiosis)[7]: The composition of a person's microbiome affects their immune system. A recent study showed that Long COVID patients had a less diverse gut microbiome than people without Long COVID. While microbiome testing isn't frequently in a gastroenterologist's toolbox, there are functional medicine tests through Genova Diagnostics and other labs that will test for dysbiosis. These tests are being conducted in research settings and can be accessed through clinical trials.

- Injury to the body from acute COVID-19 infection[8]: Since COVID-19 is not only a respiratory virus but also a systemic vascular disease,[9] it can cause an immense amount of damage to the lungs, heart, kidneys, and brain. Lasting health effects may range from long-term breathing problems and heart complications to chronic kidney impairment, stroke, and Guillain-Barré syndrome. For some patients, symptoms of Long COVID resolve when that damage is diagnosed and repaired.

- Reactivated viruses: There are many common viruses that are usually dormant in a person's body but will reawaken when the immune system is compromised from an infection.[10] These include Epstein-Barr virus (EBV), which triggers mononucleosis or "mono"; varicella-zoster, the virus that causes chickenpox and can lead to shingles; herpes simplex virus 1 (HSV-1); human herpesvirus 6 (HHV-6); and cytomegalovirus (CMV). Any doctor who is knowledgeable about post-viral illnesses— an infectious disease specialist, an immunologist, or another type of specialist—can order these tests to check for reactivations.

DIAGNOSES OF POST-VIRAL ILLNESS APPROACH

While getting to the root cause(s) of illness is ideal, it's not always feasible for people who don't have the time, money, or resources to go through the adventure of an investigation. For this reason, it's important to root your patient work in the history of infection-associated illnesses. There are common diagnoses following a virus that have been studied for far longer than SARS-CoV-2, which means you can follow the footsteps of your predecessors to an additional diagnosis. Below, we offer you information about common post-viral illnesses and comorbidities, and a framework for their diagnoses.

1. ME/CFS[11]: Myalgic encephalomyelitis—once called chronic fatigue syndrome and often abbreviated as ME/CFS—is a complex chronic disease that presents with symptoms in multiple body systems. It is a neurological disease according to the World Health Organization, and its hallmark symptom is post-exertional symptom exacerbation. While there is no one test to diagnose the condition, specialists will use tests that have shown biological abnormalities in research settings to aid in a diagnosis.

2. Dysautonomia[12]: Dysautonomia is an umbrella term for many different symptoms that can be explained by dysfunction of the autonomic nervous system. While many Long COVID patients with dysautonomia experience a spike in heart rate upon standing, dysautonomia can manifest as dizziness,

fatigue, shortness of breath, and temperature sensitivity, too. Some of the different forms of dysautonomia include postural orthostatic tachycardia syndrome (POTS) and neurocardiogenic syncope (NCS). Dysautonomia is often diagnosed by a tilt table test.

3. Mast Cell Activation Syndrome (MCAS)[13]: In MCAS, mast cell mediators are released too frequently or abundantly and/or in response to triggers that are not typically considered to be harmful, such as a food or a chemical in the environment. Inappropriately triggered inflammation leads to symptoms like difficulty breathing, hives, and low blood pressure. Diagnosis of the condition is a systematic approach, combining clinical symptoms with response to treatment, mediator tests, and ruling out other diagnoses. Tryptase is often the first mediator test used to diagnose the condition.

4. Ehlers-Danlos syndrome (EDS)[14]: EDS comprises a group of hereditary disorders of connective tissue that are varied in the ways they affect the body. They are generally characterized by joint hypermobility, joint instability, skin hyperextensibility, and other structural weaknesses. Diagnosis starts with a clinical evaluation against a set of criteria and may lead to molecular testing for confirmation.

5. Autoimmune diseases[15]: Autoimmune diseases occur when the immune system mistakenly attacks the body instead of protecting it. One of the common triggers of an autoimmune disease is infection. The diagnostic process combines lab testing, such as ANA, complete blood count (CBC), and CRP, with symptom reporting. Common autoimmune diseases include rheumatoid arthritis, systemic lupus erythematosus (lupus, SLE), Crohn's disease, psoriasis, and multiple sclerosis (MS).

Searching for or ruling out a specific post-viral diagnosis is incredibly important for you to be able to move forward as a patient. This approach, along with the Long COVID theory approach, combines the existing knowledge of the post-viral world with the developments that are continually unfolding in the Long COVID space. That being said, Long COVID is novel and unique in its presentation, and additional strange findings have cropped up everywhere. These individual findings, such as an elevated D-dimer or low vitamin D, do not paint an entire picture but can help build a story for an individual patient. Below, we offer you an outline of tests that have shown abnormalities in Long COVID patients, found either through research or patient experience.

RESEARCH-SUPPORTED BLOOD TESTS

Epstein-Barr Virus (EBV) Nuclear Antigen (EBNA)	D-Dimer
EBV Antigen-Diffuse (EA-D) IGG	Lipid Panel
EBV Viral Capsid Antigen (VCA) IGM	Iron Panel, with Ferritin
EBV VCA IGG	Homocysteine
Herpesvirus 6 (HHV-6) Antibodies (IGG, IGM)	Antinuclear Antibody (ANA)
Cytomegalovirus (CMV) Antibodies (IGG, IGM)	Complement C3 and C4
Erythrocyte Sedimentation Rate (ESR)	Rheumatoid Factor (RF)
Anticardiolipin Antibodies	Liver Function Panel with ALT & AST
Antiphospholipid Antibody Panel	Vitamin B12 (Active and Total Serum)
Immunoglobulins A (IGA), G (IgG), M (IgM)	Lactate Dehydrogenase (LDH)
Immunoglobulin G3 (IgG3)	Von Willebrand Factor (VWF)
CBC with Differential	Prothrombin Time (PT) and INR
Comprehensive Metabolic Panel (Chem20 Panel)	Glucose
TSH & Free T4	Tryptase
Full Thyroid Panel with TPO Antibodies	WBC, Neutrophils
Troponin	APTT
Vitamin D, 25- Dihydroxy	CD4 CD8 Ratio Panel (Immune System Analysis)
C-Reactive Protein (CRP)	Testosterone, Total and Free
Creatine Kinase	Follicle-Stimulating hormone (FSH)
Histamine and N-Methylhistamine	Luteinizing Hormone (LH)
Interferons: IFN-γ, IFN-α2a	Estrogen
Serum Fibrinogen Test	Progesterone
Interleukins: IL-1α, IL-1β, IL-2, IL-4, IL-5, IL-6, IL-7, IL-8, IL-10, IL-12, IL-12p70, IL-13, IL-15, IL-16, IL-17A, IL-18, IL-21, IL-33	Dehydroepiandrosterone Sulfate (DHEAS)
Tumor Necrosis Factors: TNF-α, TNF-β1	Cortisol
Vascular Endothelial Growth Factors (VEGF-A)	Natural Killer Cells, Functional
Cytokine Panel 13, Serum (inclusive of many of the interleukin levels and TNF levels cited above, however a more condensed and accessible panel for many)	Estimated Glomerular Filtration Rate (EGFR)
Apolipoprotein Evaluation	Potassium
ACE-1 and ACE-2	

PATIENT COMMUNITY-SUPPORTED BLOOD TESTS

Collagen Type II Antibodies	Eosinophils
Autoimmune Neurology Antibody Comprehensive Panel with Reflex, Serum; inclusive of Acetylcholine Receptor Ganglionic (ALPHA 3) AB	Uric Acid
Immunofluorescent Assay (IFA); Lyme Disease Reactivation Test	Adrenocorticotropic Hormone (ACTH)
Sensitive Enzyme Immunoassay (EIA); Lyme Disease Reactivation Test	Metabolomix+
IBS Differential Panel	MTFHR Gene Mutation
Phosphate	

"OTHER" SUPPORTIVE DIAGNOSTIC TESTS	
Corneal Confocal Microscopy (CCM)	Spirometry
Cardiopulmonary Exercise Testing (CPET)	Fibroscan
Cervical MRI—Craniocervical Instability (CCI)	Echo with Strain Imaging
Upright MRI (for CCI Diagnostics)	Electrocardiogram (ECG)
Oxidative Stress Analysis	Gastric Empty Study (GES)
Tilt Table Test (TTT), concurrently run with Upright Catecholamine Testing	Endothelial Function Testing
Multi-Day Portable Electrocardiogram (ECG)	10-Minute NASA Lean Test or Stand Test (Note: may take up to 30 minutes to elicit neurally mediated hypotension)
Pulmonary Peak Flow Test	Overnight Oximetry, Home Sleep Study, Polysomnography
Small Punch Skin Biopsies	

For more, visit longcovidpatient.com/diagnostics.

When even the experts don't know precisely what is happening, how do we make sense of the world into which we have suddenly been thrust as long-haulers? With every crisis comes the opportunity to make a paradigm shift. Groundbreaking COVID research and the mobilization and advocacy of patient groups have shown that much progress can be made in a short period of time. But we know that for many long-haulers, it feels like research, solutions, and time itself are creeping along. The road ahead will not be without obstacles, but we hope that we've provided some of the tools you need to actively engage with health care systems, and in doing so, to continue to uproot the systems that have historically denied you care.

Survival Tips

I. By putting in the early effort to get a diagnosis, a patient can build a strong foundation to ensure their mental health, physical health, and financial well-being are not being neglected.

- Mental health: A diagnosis helps validate the patient's experience, addresses the biological issues causing symptoms of a mental health disorder, and opens doors to (at times) comforting prognoses and support groups.

- Physical health: A diagnosis allows for discussions with physicians about treatment and symptom management, in which a patient and their provider can outline goals to inform how to move forward. Short-term goals may involve stabilizing their health to live a functional life; long-term goals require addressing the root cause of the illness while simultaneously building health.

- Financial well-being: A diagnosis unlocks medical and legal protections, such as workplace accommodations, disability income and benefits, and insurance coverage for medical costs.

2. Finding a trusted health care provider who is kind, knowledgeable, and curious is one of the most important steps to take in pursuing a diagnosis, but you can still advocate for yourself in the opposite circumstance. Questions to ask include the following:

- "What is your differential diagnosis for my condition?"
- "How have you ruled these differential diagnoses out?"
- "What is the evidence for and against that differential?"
- "Could you please document that?"

3. Depending on your situation, the framework for finding a diagnosis may differ.

- Retrieving an initial Long COVID diagnosis:
  - » Take advantage of testing (COVID-19 and other) during acute infection.
  - » Seek out antibody, T-cell, and other tests in the following weeks to validate infection.
- Finding root causes of illness:
  - » Viral persistence: Testing is mostly found in research settings.
  - » Autoimmunity: Basic testing can be ordered by a rheumatologist. More advanced testing is being done in research settings.
  - » Chronic inflammation: Basic testing can be ordered by a physician. More advanced testing is being done in research settings.
- Investigating post-viral illnesses and comorbidities:
  - » ME/CFS
  - » Dysautonomia
  - » Mast cell activation syndrome (MCAS)
  - » Ehlers-Danlos syndrome
  - » Autoimmune diseases
- Tests that have shown abnormalities in research and Long COVID patients (see above section on page 143 that outlines some tests you may pursue)

CHAPTER 7

Down in the Well, We Will Mourn and Sing

Surviving Mental Illness

Morgan Stephens

Content warning: This text contains suicidal ideation and methods.

Dear Long-Hauler,
    I wrote this chapter in the form of a letter. For something as intimate, complex, and critical as the mental health toll of Long COVID, I decided that communicating directly to you would be the best way to convey what I want you to know about Long COVID and mental health. So, here we go.

Before I got sick, I treated any mental health issue as somewhat of an afterthought, a nuisance I suppressed through achievement, a distraction to be plucked out and put aside until I had the "right time" to settle down and process what I'd been through. This was the psychological effect of being a child of parents who, by either death or divorce, came from fractured families, leaving home as a teenager to live on the other side of the country, being emotionally and financially independent at a young age, struggling as an actor in my early twenties, starting over in my mid-twenties by enrolling in a community college—and all the sacrifices and anxieties that came with that. As the years rolled on, the daily demands of life crowded out whatever anxiety and depression I had in my body, cramping it deep into a corner, where it sat to gather dust—at least that's what I thought then.

Now I realize that, throughout my life, I subconsciously used my anxiety to my benefit. It was a force that put me in a car as a teenager and drove me west. On paper, it rewarded me with a perfect grade point average and propelled me from community college to a world-renowned university. I applied my depression as fuel, a valve that stayed turned on, thrusting me forward in spite of a world that I often felt beaten down by.

Until I got sick in the winter of 2020, these parts of myself never kept me from living a full, vibrant life. It wasn't until Long COVID that I realized how much my mental health issues, and my suppression of them, affected my intentions and behavior. My abrupt deterioration from Long COVID changed this. For months, I remained in such physical and mental anguish that I didn't know if I would survive, or if I wanted to live, if this would be the quality of my life.

When you haven't slept for weeks and you're so tired, but the agitation and restlessness has you crawling in your skin. When you try to close your eyes to get some rest and you're in constant motion, the room spinning upside down and dropping as if you're on a perpetual roller coaster drop. When your fatigue and weakness force others to make your meals. When everything you fill your life with disappears—you're unable to read, write, listen to music, watch television or communicate with loved ones. When everything that made you *you* vanishes, your world becomes a dark well, tucked deep underground from the world above.

I'm not a mental health expert. I don't have all the answers—far from it. Your experience and mine, though similar in some ways, are likely different in others. That's part of what has made our illness difficult to study, diagnose, and treat. But there are commonalities that bring us together. No matter how much you try to focus on other things—on anything else at all—Long COVID grabs you by the face and holds you there, because there's nowhere else to look. It sucks you into freefall from your former life. You can't push it aside or will it away. I want to tell you that I admire your strength in getting this far against so many odds. You *will* survive Long COVID—and heal from it. This is how I got to the other side.

Recovery looks different for everyone. Some make full recoveries back to their pre-COVID selves and others have lingering symptoms years later or lifelong chronic illnesses or disabilities. I can't tell you where you'll fall, but I want you to know that you'll have support no matter what. Healing takes many forms, not just the absence of physical symptoms. We are each different and, shamefully, our socioeconomic status can affect our access to help and our ability to recover or better manage our illnesses. All I can offer is what helped—and what hurt—my progress.

As a long-hauler and a journalist, I can tell you firsthand that the mass disabling event that the COVID-19 pandemic created has also resulted in a colossal mental health crisis in which patients like you and me who desperately need help are stuck navigating a dysfunctional and bureaucratic mental health care system. However, please know that resources do exist, and there is still a way out.

First, what you're going through is unbelievably difficult and isolating—and real. You may have been questioned by people you came to in desperate need of help, or told that your symptoms stem from "anxiety" or that this is all in your head. That's what doctors, specialists, psychiatrists, chiropractors, friends, and family members often told me. I've been given diagnoses and advice that, though well-intentioned, missed the mark because they never addressed the biomedical roots and very real physical manifestations of my illness.

Second, you aren't alone; even though you might feel like it. There is a large, international community at your fingertips for any questions you might have or company you may seek. This community exists in private support groups and in the thousands of long-haulers who support one another online. This community also exists in this book. Use it as a guiding light to find tangible resources and solidarity; in reading our stories, you will join our community.

My journey started in late-November 2020. The intense suffering, both mental and physical, was unlike anything I'd ever experienced. Until March 2021, it was a fight to make it through the day. Mornings were always the worst, because their arrival meant the day was just starting. Night was best. I would feel a wave of relief when seven o'clock rolled around. That meant I had made it to the end of the day. Yet, as comforting as nighttime was, it was also a time of dread. I never knew what the long night had in store for me. Often, it meant staying awake with the intense urge to shake my body, what I now have come to know as *akathisia*, a movement disorder that makes it hard for you to stay still. Perhaps you have experienced something similar. Or maybe you've experienced vertigo, cardiac irregularities, muscle weakness, limb-swelling, post-exertional malaise, prolonged fevers, rashes or hives, psychosis, or any of the many other symptoms prevalent in our Long COVID community.

Although I'm now functional and have been able to find joy in life again, my healing journey has been a fickle road. Recovery isn't a straight line. Recognizing this was helpful for me to manage my expectations, and it may be for you, too. Some days are going to be hard—really hard. Days when your symptoms have flared after you thought you were out of the woods, when you feel the room tilt to the left from vertigo, or have to steady yourself because of breathlessness. Days when you're simply sick and tired of being sick and tired, or when you flashback and, instantly, you're in the toughest early months of your trauma, and you lay in bed sobbing and reeling in shock. It's okay to feel all of it. There will also be days that almost seem normal, where you laugh, make yourself a nice meal, have a cup of tea, and enjoy the birds chirping outside in the sun. As you begin to learn about your illness, gain support in managing it, and possibly improve, your body will come out of crisis mode.

But at the beginning, Long COVID ate me up from all sides until it caved in on everything that made up who I was. Any bit of joy dried up. The neurological symptoms that left me in a thick fog also snatched away all the ways I usually distract or console myself from pain: music, television, social media, good conversation, and reading. For months, I thought Long COVID marked the end of my life. It's not that I thought I was going to die from the disease. It's that I didn't want to live. Living with Long COVID didn't feel like living. It wasn't recovery or death—it was the limbo, the nothingness, the ghost of myself that I had to wake up and bear witness to every morning. But, slowly, I found my way back to myself, outside the limbo and back into the world of the living.

What Happened to My Brain?: Turning to the Science for Hope

According to a study released in the *Journal of the American Medical Association* (JAMA), the post-COVID brain "may resemble those involved in traumatic brain injury."[1] In March 2022, Oxford researchers discovered physical differences in the post-COVID brain, which include a reduction in gray matter and tissue damage.[2] In some of these injuries, inflammation and damage to blood vessels, which results in a loss of neurons, can heighten the risk of suicidal behavior. These researchers have described "independent brain damage" that's "unrelated to respiratory insufficiency."[3] This means that the brain damage may not in fact be a result of respiratory symptoms—which is significant because many health experts once deemed COVID only a respiratory illness. These findings instead suggest that COVID is more than a respiratory disease; it is, in fact, a neurological one as well. Other neuropsychiatric symptoms include cognitive impairment or brain fog (see chapter 8), memory loss, strokes, psychosis, and seizures.

The physical and neurological developments in my body and the changes that resulted—the end of my former life, of everything I'd worked toward—put me in a deep, dark, isolated hole. I spent days fantasizing about how I would end my suffering. I still have guilt about this. I tell you this not to frighten you, fellow long-hauler, but to be honest, so perhaps you might feel less alone if you're in a similar space or can't express how you feel to someone because you're ashamed or afraid.

If you're having thoughts of hurting yourself, planning the method of how you'll end your life, or thinking frequently about death, it's important to voice this to someone you trust. If you're having suicidal thoughts, the National Suicide Prevention hotline, 1-800-273-TALK, is there 24-7 to help. There is also a web chat feature at suicidepreventionlifeline.org/chat.

According to the CDC, one in five Americans experience Long COVID.[4] Other studies have estimated prevalence in a similar range, but more research is needed. It is likely that tens of millions of Americans are affected.[5] That means around seventeen million Americans, as of this writing, will be dealing with Long COVID. Some neurological dysfunction may be related to inflammation in the brain[6] from the immune response to the virus or the virus itself. Long COVID patients are at a heightened risk of suicide. I won't bore you with all of the science, but, in short, researchers have confirmed that COVID can affect the structure of the blood-brain barrier, beginning a cascade that can impair learning and memory.[7] This neurological impact can manifest as mental health issues. Yes, Long COVID is in your head, but not in the way gaslighting skeptics might believe. *It's actually in your brain.*

I know this is scary. Early on, I was terrified. I kept thinking that my intellect and indefatigable drive made me who I was. Reading, writing, communicating, and tossing around ideas on complex issues in politics, public policy, and social justice were why I became a journalist. For a few months, I lost all of this. It was devastating, but because I could barely make it through the day, I didn't have it in me to address the potentially colossal loss of all I'd worked toward for half a decade. I was in survival mode. There was no time to worry about the faults or benefits in tax deductions, climate change mitigation policies, or presidential appointments.

It hit home on January 6, 2021, when the Capitol Hill insurrection occurred. That day, I sat in a daze, staring blankly at the TV. The screen hurt my eyes, and I couldn't comprehend what was happening. My husband, Jerry, glanced over at me, looking for hints of my former self to emerge—interested, ignited, angry. Instead, I looked away, my mother turned off the TV, and my husband crept back upstairs.

Happily, and as you can tell, I'm writing again. I can listen to music, watch television, and communicate with others. I can sleep. I can walk to the Long Beach harbor and smell the salty, ocean air. I can find joy in hugging my sweet dog. I can strategize again, play cards, and plan. My brain has healed enough to do these things. Despite the many dark moments, you can also find moments of hope.

When I got sick, I tried to read articles about neuroplasticity. Until the 1960s, neurologists thought the brain couldn't heal after infancy and childhood.[8] But more recent medical discoveries have shown that brains are adaptive and can heal even in adults.[9] It's an ongoing process in which the brain can reorganize itself, both structurally in its ability to make new neural pathways and functionally in its ability to move function from a damaged area to an undamaged one. If you're experiencing decreased brain function, you can work with a brain specialist on exercises that target remapping and growth, at a safe pace that doesn't trigger any relapses.

For me, it was like a flipped switch. One day I was fine, and the next, something was terribly wrong. It was as if I'd been given a stimulant, like an electric current that caused me to feel restless along with a heavy sense of doom and dread. I felt like I was cloaked in a ten-pound blanket. One morning in late January 2021, Jerry and I went to the grocery store. By the time we'd made our way to the checkout counter, I couldn't hold myself up any longer. I braced myself by grabbing onto the conveyor belt and asked him for the keys. Exhausted, I sat in the car while he finished paying.

When we got home, this feeling of exhaustion, mixed with the restlessness I'd been feeling for months, propelled me outside to our back deck, where I hurled myself onto the ground. My limp body lay there, my face pressing against the cold wood in the chilly air.

"What the hell are you doing?" Jerry asked, startled, when he saw the back door open and me lying outside in the cold. He walked over, crouched down, and said, "C'mon, get up." I just stared.

Many people won't understand why we do the things we do while we are ill. Sometimes, I don't fully understand it. Was throwing myself onto the deck my feeble and irrational attempt to throw myself out of my body? Was it that the shock of the cold air brought with it an openness, when our heated four-wall home felt like it was closing in on me? I'm still not sure.

I won't psychologize our illness. We've experienced plenty of that. But I will tell you what it looks like to be psychologized. In early December 2020, just after I fell ill, I started to keep a symptom journal. But when I'd try to describe my long list of bizarre symptoms to my doctors, I'd sense the room change.

"I'm having, like, brain zaps, and hallucinations. I've felt as if photos on the wall were threatening," I'd say, "I feel like I'm spinning upside down, I have adrenaline-like restlessness and a feeling that I need to shake my body." The doctor and nurse would exchange looks. It was clear they questioned my story, and it was devastating that, at my most vulnerable, the people who were supposed to help me gaslit me instead.

I knew how it looked from the outside. The longer my symptom list got, the more unstable I began to look. As time went on, I became conditioned not to mention any of my symptoms that made me look like I'd lost it. But, dear long-hauler, I don't want you to do this. Even if they won't listen, tell them. If someone can't look outside their purview, that's their problem, not yours. Don't give up on finding health care providers who will listen, who acknowledge all they may not know, and who are committed to trying to help you. That being said, I know you will face barriers. You might feel tossed aside or viewed as if it's all in your head. Know that I have felt that, too.

In the months shortly after I got sick, I was diagnosed with a multitude of psychological diagnoses, ranging from generalized anxiety disorder and major depressive disorder to bipolar disorder—all triggered by this illness. This trauma cannot be erased. I will carry it with me. You likely do or will, too. In that way, we're bound—to one another, and to tens of millions of others. We implicitly understand one another because our illness and the trauma it causes is so often invisible. We know the strange, indescribable, palpable dread, the electric feeling that pulls at the bottom of our throats, the fog that keeps us from being able to make a meal or remember what day it is, the insomnia that keeps us moving from room to room as our families sleep, the internal tremors that nobody can see but that feel as if an earthquake is underneath us, the fatigue that makes getting a book out of a drawer an impossible task and keeps us chained to our beds. These are the scars nobody else can see. They bond us. And those bonds are deep, intimate, and lasting.

There may be roadblocks ahead, from long wait times for psychologists and psychiatrists to the risk of suicide. In 2019, the average wait time to see a mental health provider was twenty-five days, with one in five psychiatrists not seeing new patients.[10] Now, with the new, large swath of patient demand, that number is even smaller.[11] Depressive symptoms have increased threefold during the pandemic, with those in lower socioeconomic brackets at greater risk.[12] Due to immense loss, lockdowns, and economic stress, providers are unable to meet the demand for patient care. If we consider the tens of millions of people who will seek care for neurological and mental illness caused by COVID-19, the situation becomes more extreme. And those are just the confirmed case numbers. My family, and so many other families I've spoken with, have been left to navigate it alone. Some have experienced devastating consequences, with a family member suffering with Long COVID symptoms attempting or dying by suicide. This reinforces that Long COVID is a mental health crisis of epic proportions.

If you are insured, try to find a mental health care provider in your area who is taking new patients, and if you're uninsured, try to find a subsidized program (a simple Google search should bring up a variety of sources in your area) that takes patients. I'll list a few specific options on page 158 that you may find helpful. But I recognize that finding help is often easier said than done. I've seen firsthand how dysfunctional our health care system is in providing accessibility in times of crisis. We need more funding, more resources, and more psychologists and psychiatrists to meet the demand. This book, with tangible resources marked in every chapter, can be a starting point to help you get through it.

How Do I Get Help? Finding Health Care Providers and Counselors

Mental health resources are important to get through the worst days and, once you've crossed over out of crisis mode, to support healing. Living with the aftermath of a virus that can leave you in a perpetual state of illness and exhaustion, makes depression, anxiety, and post-traumatic stress disorder (PTSD) seem all but unavoidable. PTSD is a "trauma and stress" disorder. DSM-5, a guide used for clinicians to diagnose mental health disorders, states that signs of PTSD can present as flashbacks, where the individual feels as if the trauma is recurring and experiences intrusive memories, hypervigilance, intense or prolonged distress, avoidance of stimuli associated with the trauma, inability to remember an important aspect of the trauma, reactions to internal or external cues that resemble the trauma, and feelings of detachment or estrangement from others.[13] Applied to Long COVID patients, complex post-traumatic stress disorder (C-PTSD) accounts for the *duration* of the trauma.

In the early nineties, Harvard University researcher Dr. Judith Herman found that C-PTSD was a syndrome of "prolonged and repeated trauma,"[14] which applies to many people living with Long COVID. Symptoms include behavioral changes like impulsivity, self-destructive behavior, drug and alcohol misuse, emotional difficulties like rage, depression, and panic, and cognitive difficulties like dissociation and derealization. Often, C-PTSD can inhibit our desire or ability to continue to seek care.

"I think I'm in shock about what's happening," I blurted out to my mother from the passenger seat on the way home from yet another doctor's visit. We'd gone looking for answers but had received none. I sobbed, softly through the thick haze. I laid the seat all the way back and stared out at the gray sky through the car windows. Before that appointment during the first weeks I became ill, my mother spent hours each day setting up appointments with clinics. But, by then, it felt like a lost cause. The swift, deep heartbreak I carried from the abrupt decline of my physical and mental health had cast me into a kind of shell shock. As the months passed, the rides home became quieter. The air inside the car, heavier. This heaviness blew into the house as we opened the door, with nothing to tell my awaiting father and husband. Eventually, we stopped looking to doctors to find answers.

It's important to acknowledge the deep emotional wounds and PTSD that are caused by living with a chronic, not-well-understood illness, as well as the medical gaslighting that we've been exposed to at our most vulnerable. If you identify with these symptoms, I recommend you give yourself time to process what you're feeling and hold space for those emotions. You can also reach out to support groups to discuss what you're feeling or seek talk therapy to work through it.

Here's what helped me. Have an advocate, like a friend or family member to join you during doctor's appointments, especially if you are in a cognitively impaired state. The more voices advocating on your behalf in the room, the better. Access to therapy and prescription medication is a vital *part* of the solution. It's not the whole solution, of course. We know we need treatment to repair the damage to our bodies from COVID-19, but since *neurological sequelae* (neurological symptoms that persist after your acute infection) affect *neuronal activity* (how your brain functions to make and maintain neurological connections), people with Long COVID can experience serotonin and dopamine irregularity or even psychosis. Prescription medication can keep us in the game and stabilize us while we go through the worst of it.

Remember that resources are there. Our approaches to mental health, disability, and chronic illness in the US are flawed; we have a long way to go. Long COVID gave me an up-close glimpse into these systemic and cultural failures. Public policy, insurance companies, and health care providers have long failed to make mental health care quick to access and affordable to the majority of Americans. A 2018 study by Cohen Veterans Network revealed that lack of access was the root cause of the mental health crisis in the US[15]—and this was before the pandemic increased the demand for mental health services. This lack of access was a result of high cost and insufficient insurance coverage, long wait times, lack of awareness or not knowing where to go, and social stigma.

You may be afraid of being judged as "weak" or "crazy" for being open about depression or anxiety or other neuropsychiatric symptoms like paranoia and hallucinations. It takes great strength to come forward and be open in a society that has historically stigmatized these topics. But we're moving in the right direction, as more people are starting to share their mental health struggles. So, know that if or when you are ready to share your experience, there will be a community there to support you. Even if you face these barriers, I still recommend reaching out for help. If your current mental capacity makes it too difficult, ask a friend, family member, or support group member to help you.

Since the demand for care is high and waitlists are long, you may want to consider websites and apps that offer virtual therapy like BetterHelp, Cerebral, and Talkspace, which offer services with licensed therapists through video conferencing, phone, or online messaging. This could be a good option if you don't have insurance or reliable transportation or if you work unconventional hours. At the time of this writing, BetterHelp starts at $240 a month and goes up to $600, depending on your geographic location. Talkspace is a subscription-based service, starting at $65 per week or $240 per month and accepts some insurances. Cerebral takes insurance and is similar to other competitors' prices and services.

There are also federal resources from the National Institute of Mental Health, like the Health Resources and Services Administration (HRSA). They can work with you to find affordable health care in your area with sliding scale rates. The 1-800-662-HELP hotline to the Substance Abuse and Mental Health Services Administration (SAMHSA) can get you answers to general mental health questions and help you locate services in your area. National agencies and nonprofits like the Anxiety and Depression Association of America, Mental Health America, and the National Alliance on Mental Health can help you find mental health services and information on mental health conditions and policy in the US.

Be sure to pace yourself when reading information about Long COVID. Of course, discussing your mental health with your health care provider and staying updated on Long COVID research is important. But you may need to take breaks. As I went deeper down the rabbit hole of doom, reading journal articles and trying to comprehend, in my impaired state, all that could go wrong in post-COVID patients, I realized this was a double-edged sword.

On one hand, familiarizing myself with the latest medical journal articles and research on my illness brought me a sense of control and comfort. You can bring the journal articles to your health care appointments or send them via message so your doctors are up to speed (for more on how to use research to help you, see chapter 11). The way I felt, especially in late 2020 when I was spiraling out of control, was that if I wasn't going to try to figure it out, then who was? I was frustrated that nobody seemed capable of helping, yet I was so determined to understand what was happening to my body that I spent hours desperately parsing through jargon-filled medical reports.

On the other hand, knowing what could continue to go wrong wasn't always helpful for my mental health, and I often discovered after my long research sessions that I hadn't actually taken in much information, because my brain fog was so severe. The more I dug into the medical reports and studies, the more my brain, already in a state of fight or flight, felt that anxiety and dread.

Finding balance is key. Familiarize yourself with post-viral illnesses like ME/CFS and POTS, stress responses like PTSD and C-PTSD, and some of the literature that might point to answers about your condition. But don't bombard yourself. If you start feeling overwhelmed by the information or convinced your life is spiraling to a point of no return, try taking a break. Taking even a few moments to care for yourself and do something that makes you happy can make all the difference. At the very least, it can simply get you to tomorrow.

Am I Really Alone in This? Long COVID Is a Family Affair

In late January, after a month of seeing over a dozen doctors who didn't have respect for my pain or didn't believe me, I stopped seeking answers. I was playing a game of trial and error to see which antidepressants and which vertigo and sleep medications I responded to best. These experiments with medications caused additional side effects, and it was often hard to tell what was a result of a medication not working and what was my brain misfiring. It became difficult for me to communicate. But Long COVID was affecting more than just me—it was impacting my family, too.

Content warning: This section contains suicidal ideation and methods. To skip this section, turn to page 163.

I'm including an account of my suicidal ideation and how close Long COVID brought me to death in the hope that, by sharing it, you may feel less alone in your own struggle. If you happen to go down this dark road, too, I'm here to say, *hold on.* You will get past this. If you think reading the details of my story may be triggering, I encourage you to flip to page 163.

In the winter of 2020, when I wasn't sleeping and felt as if my brain was operating in a post-concussive state, I sunk into a deep depression. Because of the long waits for mental health services, it took two months for me to be able to see a psychiatrist.

I knew something was cognitively off when, about a week after the fog set in, in early December, as I lay in bed with my mother watching TV, I made a silent pact with myself that if I got worse, I would kill myself. This thought brought me an instant wave of relief. I should've told someone, but I didn't. I didn't want to frighten my family. I knew they'd immediately try to get me help, and that would mean hospital stays and psychiatric evaluations. Those fears eventually came true anyway, when the suicidal ideation got worse and I couldn't hide it any longer. Eventually I accepted that I would end my life; I just had to do it in the least painful way possible, to make it easier for both myself and my family.

At the end of December, my mother tried, in vain, to calm me. She tried to remind me that life might be worth living, and when my insomnia just wouldn't quit, she brought me to the ocean. She booked a suite at a Hilton, right by the beach—only a four-hour drive away. I've loved the ocean since I was a child. When I was young, we spent summers on the coast vacationing as a family, making sandcastles; when I got older, I swam in the sea, letting the salty, sandy water dampen my lemon-juice-soaked hair as my friends and I giggled and glanced over at the boys floating on their bodyboards.

Mom and I settled into our twenty-fourth-floor suite, but when night came, she slept and I stayed awake, shaking. "Will I continue to deteriorate until I'm no longer able to make my own decisions?" Relief beckoned me. I walked to the balcony and opened the sliding glass door. A rush of salty, cool wind blew through my hair as I stared over the edge—*a long way down.* Then, instinctively, I stepped back, thinking about the weight my family would carry for the rest of their lives if I made the jump. I closed the door and got back into bed. When the sun came up, my mother sat next to me and held my hand in bed as I writhed.

"How'd you sleep?" she asked.

"Why won't God just let me go?" I moaned. "Let me die."

By now I was angry. I was angry that my body had betrayed me, angry at the suffering I was forced to endure each long day and night, angry at everything I had so carefully crafted for my life, that was now out of sight in a matter of weeks.

She drove me straight to the hospital.

"She keeps saying she's ready to go—to die," my mother interjected in the ER exam room.

The ER doctor glanced over at me and asked if I had thoughts about ending my life. In my gut, I felt a swift reflex of defensiveness. I knew what happened in hospitals when you told them you didn't want to live anymore.

I lowered my eyes.

Then, I said it: "I don't want to die, but if you felt this way, you wouldn't want to live either. I'm in agony! My quality of life is horrible."

I started quietly sobbing.

"She's been wanting to go to Belgium. For an assisted suicide," Mom said.

The doctor told me she understood my plight, but hospital protocol required me to see a psychiatrist before they would discharge me. I was immediately assigned a nurse, who kept her eyes on me, sitting at the door to make sure I didn't escape. She offered me scratchy blue scrubs and yellow hospital socks with rubber stoppers in exchange for my clothing, my cell phone, and my wedding ring, which she instructed me to place in a large plastic bag. Due to the hospital's suicide protocol, she asked that I change into the scrubs with the door open. They wheeled me out of the room as two police officers kept watch to make sure I didn't run out of the hospital. If I did, they were there to detain me. They deposited me into a windowless white cement brick room overnight, to wait to speak to the in-house psychiatrist, who had left the night before at 10 PM.

After I begged for them, the nurse found me some ear plugs to drown out the incessant piercing beeps coming from the machines in the ER. I was still so sensitive to light and sound. At home, every noise—from the television, the ticking of the clock, a guided meditation—was painful and anxiety-provoking. These loud machines were so much worse.

The next morning, a nurse walked in and turned on the fluorescent lights. I covered my eyes to dampen the sharp pain of the brightness. She wheeled a desk with a computer to the foot of my bed. A few clicks later, I heard a man's voice.

When I sat up and looked at the screen, I felt like metal corkscrews were twisting into my brain. The man was on the screen, sitting in what looked like a home office; he was middle-aged, with a balding head and brown goatee, wearing a small pair of glasses. He asked me a few general questions about myself to gauge how much I was in, or out of, touch with reality and my cognitive impairment, like "What day is it?" which I'm sure I didn't remember, "What year is it?" which I did remember, and "Who is the president?" I answered correctly: "Donald Trump." When he asked about sleep, I told him I hadn't slept in over a month.

Then, he got to the goods.

"Do you have thoughts about harming yourself?"

"Yes," I moaned, looking down at the cold, white laminated floors, running my fingers through strands of hair.

"Do you have thoughts about harming others?"

"No. God, no."

"Do you have plans to harm yourself?"

"No . . . I just want to feel better. I'm sick."

"If you go home, do you promise not to harm yourself?

"Yes."

He prescribed me a potent sleep aid and the morning ER doctor discharged me. When they gave my clothes back and said I was free to go, all I heard was, "your sentence was pardoned." I'll never forget how that felt. I didn't wait to change out of my scrubs. I just wanted out.

"Get me the *hell* out of here," I barked, loud enough for the new nurse on-watch in my hospital room doorway to hear. I dashed past him, through the parking lot, and toward my mother's car, the scratchy blue scrubs fluttering against the freezing morning air.

The new sleep medication didn't help any of my other Long COVID symptoms, and it didn't eliminate my suicidal thoughts. But it got me to sleep five hours a night—a victory at that point. Unfortunately, this still wasn't enough. In my impaired state, I felt angry that my family wouldn't let me kill myself. For months, I continued to beg my parents to take me to Belgium for an assisted suicide.

"I'm in pain!" I'd moan and writhe in my olive green three-day-worn pajamas. I'd lost so much weight due to my lack of appetite that they were starting to hang off me. "I'm suffering," I'd cry. "You have to promise me that if I don't get better, you'll let me go."

"I will not promise you that," my brokenhearted mother said. By then, she'd lost the bright sparkle in her eyes. A dull emptiness had washed over them.

In the winter of 2020 and early 2021, as my family and I waited for the sun to set, each day buoying us to the next, my thoughts of assisted suicide became less frequent. A few months later, as the spring brought some warm sunshine to my face, and my symptoms slowly—very slowly—began to improve, I regained some function. All of a sudden, I was looking backward. I saw those crushing days had added up to weeks, then months. And, I didn't fully realize it, but I had somehow crawled out of the dark. For months I had dreaded the passage of time, but time eventually healed me.

How Can I Find a Way Out?: Support Groups Can Be a Lifeline

This brings me to my next roadblock—isolation and loneliness—and a crucial resource that helped me: support groups. Long COVID can be so isolating. My advice, dear long-hauler, is to find your people. It doesn't matter where; just look for others with similar experiences. If you look for them, they'll be there.

After months of feeling hopeless, I remembered someone we had booked on the CNN show I was working on before I got sick. She was an administrator of a support group, who spoke bravely about her neurological issues that stemmed from her COVID-19 infection in an interview on August 6, 2020. Her name was Hannah Davis. At this point, it was December, and I was experiencing the very symptoms she had described. So, I reached out to her on Twitter. I knew I was blurring the line between news professional and source. But, as the days went on, I was moving further away from the consummate professional I'd been, deeper into the land of the unwell.

Hannah responded right away. She sent me an invite to the private Long COVID support group she helped run on Slack. I logged in and immediately saw thousands of posts about what I was experiencing. There were specific channels on symptoms like neurological issues or dysautonomia (see chapter 2), links to studies, a channel for recent news, and a specific forum for supplement advice.

There was even a mental health channel for questions, and a "venting" channel for when I needed to release loneliness and frustration. This community of people with shared experiences, ready to lift one another up, was pivotal in getting me through the toughest days. While I was physically alone suffering with Long COVID, this group made it so I knew I was never actually alone, and neither are you. Many days, I communicated through severe brain fog, sleep deprivation, and restlessness.

In January 2021, I saw that there were support group members that met regularly over Zoom. One really bad day, I logged on. I'd never felt so vulnerable. Many of them were "first-wavers" infected with the virus in March of 2020, who could offer me, a "second-waver," advice and hope from their own experiences. The moment we started speaking to each other, I knew it had been a good decision to join. "I'm having horrible thoughts," I admitted one day. "I don't know if I want to live anymore, not like this."

The voices of these strangers immediately jumped in to help. One person told me that they, too, had had those thoughts at one point and that it got better. Then more people spoke up. After each person shared their story with me, they reminded me that I wouldn't feel like this forever, and to hold on.

Today, the "regulars" in that group are dear friends, or rather, as we say, "war buddies." I speak to them weekly, and we talk about our progress and setbacks. When the only thing we had was one another and my only focus was to survive to see another day, I knew there was always a lifeline. All I had to do was log on and hear a familiar voice.

All of their stories validated my experience and served as a testament to survival of the illness. And they were right. I did survive it. You will, too.

Our bodies might've betrayed us, but we never betrayed one another.

Celebrating Small Victories as
We Climb Out of the Dark

One of the unfortunate truths about our illness is that we can't exactly return to our old vibrant and healthy lives in a snap. It's a slog. But if I look back to where I was then and where I am now, the healing has been substantial. I got there with tiny steps. Steps that, to a non–chronically ill person, might be seen as ordinary and basic human tasks. Yet, I, and those around me, knew they were monumental achievements.

It started with making my own cups of tea. Well, it started with finding a sleep-aiding medication, after much trial and error, that helped me sleep at least six hours each night. This was a major victory for me after coming out of two months of severe sleep deprivation, and my body slowly started to come out of crisis mode. One day, instead of Jerry bringing me my breakfast, I staggered to the cabinet, pulled out a mug, and brewed my own tea. I went back to bed in my dizzy fog, then drank it. Soon, I began to tolerate coffee again. We both celebrated the "smallest" joys as if we had just achieved something huge. A ritual as simple as sipping piping hot coffee from my favorite mug in the morning felt like I'd been given a slice of joy back.

My next achievement was baths. I began to feel capable of running my own baths, pouring the lavender bath salts in, soaking, then getting myself out, picking out my pajamas, and getting dressed on my own without Mom's or Jerry's help. Sometimes, I'd end up taking two or three baths in a row, because they helped pass the time and brought me momentary relief from the physical pain, despair, and restlessness. In an occupational therapy session focused on self-care and pacing (see chapter 3), I joked about my inclination to take more than one bath a day.

In her professional expertise and wisdom, my therapist said, "You're healing. If you want two baths, take two baths. If you feel like you need permission, just think of me saying it's okay."

So, if you, too, want to take two baths, here is your permission. If you want to listen to the same comforting song on repeat, drive around your town aimlessly, binge-watch trash TV, or stare at the smoke from incense wafting through your space in silence, that's okay. I've learned to be less critical of myself, and to honor what brings me moments of joy, no matter how small or "weird." As we heal, if that's all we have to get us through, then that's what we have. As time passes, these moments of joy are no longer as fleeting.

This doesn't minimize the debilitation our illness inflicts on our life. Long COVID is a loss of innocence, a life turned abruptly on its head, a hard lesson that sometimes a turn of events can bring you to your knees, or that everything you've worked toward can disappear for no reason. Even with these hard truths, there is solace. You have a community that will mourn with you. I decided early on to measure my progress not in days, weeks, or even months but in three-month periods. I'd look back after three months and really see how much more I was capable of, how much more joy I was taking in. On good days, you'll laugh about silly things with friends—maybe even new friends who share your illness experience. You might even develop a dark sense of humor, like I have, finding amusement in the absurdity of how seriously I used to take my five- and ten-year goals, how rigid my plan for my life was, and how I was convinced that I needed to take specific steps to succeed.

Know that you're not alone; I offer you community and permission to be sad, devastated, confused, or angry—like really fucking angry—some days. Then, I encourage you to exhale through the glints of light and peace, and to enjoy the tiny pleasures that you find out really aren't all that tiny, like hot baths, clean bed sheets, the warmth of the sun, or the moment of pure love that you feel as you grasp a loved one's hand in yours.

We can strike a balance, surrender, *and* be active in our quest for healing. When I talk about healing, I mean finding peace, fulfillment, and a semblance of normalcy in life again outside of crisis mode. This looks different for each long-hauler. I've come to terms with the fact that I'm a passenger—in my illness and in my life. This act of surrender, in pre-COVID times, would have left me feeling helpless. Now, it's incredibly freeing. I have my toolbox to keep me above water. Don't minimize these tools; lean into them.

You might think, in this silence, this lack of acknowledgment from public health officials, that the world is "moving on." You might grieve and rage at the nature of your illness in its cruel invisibility. You might despair that you've been forgotten. At times, these fears dragged me back into that dark well. But as much as you might feel stuck there, remember that wells are also a source of supply, of nourishment and resource. You haven't been forgotten—not by me and not by the millions of other people like you. Together, our brittle, broken voices are getting louder. And, in unison, they'll sing out. We'll get the help we so desperately need and deserve.

I know you'll find relief and healing, albeit slowly, and in your own ways. In the meantime, take care of yourself, whatever that looks like for you. And when it gets dark, as it sometimes does, you might return to the essentials of what makes life worth living. Tonight, I'll put on my headphones and listen to Jeff Buckley and Elizabeth Fraser sing "All Flowers in Time Bend Towards the Sun." His hopeful falsetto will sink into my bones and carry me toward tomorrow.

Survival Tips

1. You're not alone. There's a community of other long-haulers here for you through various platforms online (see more in chapter 10).

2. Don't be afraid to ask for help. It's okay to be angry. It's okay to be sad. It's okay to *not be okay*. But please know that it gets better, and that there are people who want to and can help.

3. Long COVID may cause suicidal ideation. There's still a lot of science to be done on the neurological and neuropsychiatric effects of Long COVID. However, the little research we have shows that changes in the brain may include a reduction in gray matter and tissue damage—either due to inflammation or damage in the blood vessels. This can lead to suicidal ideation.

4. Keep a symptom journal to bring with you to health care provider's appointments. Tell your doctor what you're experiencing, no matter how scary or uncomfortable it may feel. This leaves a paper trail if you have to apply for disability later.

5. Involve others. Be it family or friends, gather support from people you trust. If possible, bring someone with you to health care appointments as an advocate.

6. Long COVID can be a traumatic experience. Becoming familiar with PTSD and C-PTSD can be helpful in recognizing patterns and behaviors, knowing how to identify them, and working with them and seeking care.

7. Finding the right medication regimen with a health care provider and going to talk therapy can be crucial to your mental health. Since the demand is high and waitlists are long, websites and apps that offer virtual therapy like BetterHelp, Cerebral, and Talkspace, can provide help while you wait. They offer services with licensed therapists through video conferencing, phone, or online messaging.

8. Celebrate small victories. If you weren't able to go for a walk but you made yourself a cup of coffee all on your own, that's a victory. If you spent the morning paying a bill then rested for the remainder of the day, that's a victory.

9. Avoid measuring progress in days or weeks. Measuring your progress every three-months can be helpful to keep a balanced perspective and accept the (often annoyingly) slow nature of Long COVID healing.

10. Simple, small joys are not so small after all. Things like taking a hot bath, doing a meditation, talking on Zoom to a support group or on the phone to a friend, watering the plants, or going for a mindful walk can make a big difference. Honor these fleeting moments without any gains or goals in sight, enjoying them for what they are—nothing more, nothing less. You'll see that this can help you get to the other side.

CHAPTER 8

Am I Making Any Sense?

Navigating Cognitive Dysfunction

Terri L. Wilder, MSW, and Yochai Re'em, MD

Terri L. Wilder, MSW, is an award-winning social worker, writer, and activist focused on disability justice for people living with HIV, Long COVID, and myalgic encephalomyelitis (ME). She was diagnosed with ME in March 2016. Terri was finishing her PhD in sociology at Georgia State University when she became ill in 2014; however, she believes she has had the disease since 1996. Since her diagnosis she has worked with elected officials, public health departments, health care providers, and activists across the globe. She is currently a consultant with #MEAction and has represented the organization on the federal Chronic Fatigue Syndrome Advisory Committee (CFSAC). She uses the skills she has learned from the AIDS movement and the LGBTQ community to fight for the ME/CFS and Long COVID community. Terri is also a journalist with TheBodyPro (thebodypro.com), a website founded in 2002 to support the HIV/AIDS workforce.

Yochai Re'em, MD, is a psychiatrist and psychotherapist whose personal experience with Long COVID in 2020 led him to seek answers outside of traditional medical systems. After a month of confusion over ongoing symptoms that included gastrointestinal and neuromuscular issues, Yochai connected with the Patient-Led Research Collaborative, and began working with them to conduct a large international survey on Long COVID. Their study was the first to systematically describe the timeline of symptoms in the first six months of Long COVID. Yochai's research and personal experience with the disease also led him to become interested in treating individuals with Long COVID who were experiencing psychological or psychiatric difficulties. While Yochai himself didn't experience significant cognitive symptoms as a part of his Long COVID experience, his research and work with patients experiencing brain fog, among other Long COVID symptoms, have informed the conversation in this chapter.

This chapter will discuss aspects related to cognitive dysfunction, or brain fog, as a component of Long COVID and ME/CFS. We've chosen to present our chapter as a transcribed conversation, because it was more accessible for Terri, whose brain fog precludes her from being able to sit and write long text. Considering that Long COVID is relatively new, and there is much emerging evidence suggesting many similarities between ME/CFS and Long COVID, we elected to focus on Terri's experience with cognitive dysfunction as it relates to ME/CFS, with the hope that readers will be able to learn from her experience and apply it to their own.

The transcript has been edited for brevity and clarity.

Yochai Re'em: Why don't we start with talking about the time in your life when you first realized that you were experiencing brain fog or cognitive dysfunction. Tell me a little bit about what it was like—did you know that it was cognitive dysfunction? Did you think it was something else? How has your experience evolved since then?

Terri Wilder: It's one of the issues that I think I have the most challenges around. I'm thinking back—I was diagnosed with myalgic encephalomyelitis in 2016, but I should tell you about when it really came to my attention. I started my PhD program in 2005, and it was supposed to be done by 2015. Around 2014, I remember thinking *something's not shooting right with my brain. I'm not tracking conversations.* I would be in the middle of a conversation, and I couldn't remember what we were talking about or I couldn't retrieve a word that I knew was on the tip of my tongue. I couldn't work on my dissertation, because things wouldn't go from my brain to my fingertips on my laptop. I thought, *I'm in my late forties, I'm getting closer to fifty. Maybe this is what happens.*

Yochai: You tried to normalize it.

Terri: I totally tried to normalize it and justify it. I wondered: *Am I becoming dumber?* But I'm not a stupid person. I've always been successful in school and work. *What is happening? Is my brain melting?* It wasn't until I got diagnosed with ME/CFS in March of 2016 that it all made sense.

Cognitive dysfunction is a key symptom for diagnosis in many of the clinical criteria for myalgic encephalomyelitis. Once I read the Institute of Medicine's 2015 diagnostic criteria for ME/CFS, I started looking things up and connecting with other people with ME, and hearing their stories. *This was common.* That's when I really realized.

Yochai: And you were at the tail end of your PhD program.

Terri: Correct, and that's stress time. You've got to churn out that dissertation and you really have to zone in and concentrate and use your analytical skills and critical thinking skills, and I just couldn't get the words out.

Yochai: ME/CFS is something that most people have never heard of—in fact, probably most doctors actually haven't heard about it or don't know much about it. How did you go about getting that diagnosis, finding someone who was able to give it to you?

Terri: It's not just doctors—most people who work in the medical care field don't know much about it.

I have a long history in working in HIV, and I'm very close with a famous AIDS activist named Peter Staley. He posted on his social media a picture of him sitting on a panel next to a woman. When I asked him who she was, he said she doesn't work in HIV; she has this other disease and she's making a documentary. So, I clicked on her name—it was Jen Brea—and that took me to #MEAction's website. I started reading, and I literally picked up the phone and called Peter, and said, "Holy shit—I have what she has."

Yochai: Wow, so you diagnosed yourself, really.

Terri: Essentially, yeah. I've heard from others that self-diagnosing is very common because there are so few health care providers with knowledge and training on this disease. So, people are forced to be their own private investigators to try to figure out what's going on with their bodies. I realize health care providers frown on "Dr. Google," but educating yourself online can be helpful sometimes. I should also note that I've had certain advantages navigating this disease. It helped that I was somewhat familiar with the medical world, which led to me being taken more seriously.

Right after I learned about Jen and ME/CFS, I found out she was coming to New York City, where I live, for an event, and I reached out and asked her if she could meet. We had a three-hour meeting. I remember it being so hard to communicate with her because my brain wasn't working. All through the conversation, I kept saying, "Am I making sense? Did you follow what I just said?"

At the end of our meeting, she said, "I am not a doctor, but you sound like you have ME." I said, "Great, what do I do? What pill do I take?" Looking back, this is laughable, because I wish there was a pill we could take. So, she gave me a couple of names of medical providers in New York City and I called the first two. They didn't take insurance.

So, I ended up with the physician that I saw because she took my health insurance. I was so sick the day that I went for my first appointment, I could barely hail a cab. I was in a—we call it a crash or post-exertional malaise (PEM).

When I got to the office, the physician said, "Just looking at you, I can tell you are so sick. I cannot believe you're working." And I told her I could barely make it to work and back. I would go to work, come home, and get in bed. I would pray to make it to Friday because then I knew I could be in bed from Friday evening to Monday morning. I was so, so sick.

Yochai: What were you doing for work at that time?

Terri: I worked at Mount Sinai Hospital. They have an HIV program and I was the director of HIV education and training.

And interestingly, my grant that was funded through the New York State Department of Health was for training medical providers on HIV and Hepatitis C and LGBTQ+ health. So, I have a long history in the medical world, and I understand how the medical system works. I was shocked when I got diagnosed with a disease that . . . apparently nobody cares about.

Yochai: And it sounds like your job at the time required a fair amount of cognitive effort.

Terri: Yeah, and it was a real struggle. I almost had this kind of imposter syndrome. "How do I keep up the appearance that I'm capable, and nothing's changed, and I'm on top of my work and managing my team and meeting my deliverables?" It was a struggle to get everything done on time at the quality that was expected, all while I felt like my brain was melting. I was really grieving my brain.

Yochai: Tell me more about the brain fog symptoms. You talked about the thoughts in your head not getting translated to your fingertips while working on the dissertation. What else was part of the brain fog?

Terri: Word retrieval was an issue. I often couldn't find the words I wanted to say, sometimes in the middle of a conversation. It was harder for me to write sentences, like putting the words in order or making the paragraphs flow for the main point. I also work for a very large HIV website, and I used to write news articles for them. I approached the editor, whom I have a very long good relationship with, and I told him I couldn't write articles anymore. But I asked him if there was something that we could figure out, because I get so much fulfillment out of this work. We ended up reaching an agreement where I could do recorded interviews with people about HIV-related topics, and we would transcribe and edit them. That allowed me to still make a contribution, still make some money.

Sometimes, I didn't understand what people were saying to me. I couldn't receive the message that they were conveying in a sentence. I would say, "I'm sorry, what are you trying to say? What does that mean?"

I was also having memory issues. I would watch a movie and then a few weeks later I would watch it again, and I wouldn't realize that I had already seen it until later. The cognitive issues have just kind of been all over the place for me, but I will say that they are at their worst when I'm in a crash. My guess would be that that's pretty common for people who have cognitive dysfunction—that it's worse when they're in a crash or in the middle of post-exertional malaise.

Yochai: And when you finally found a doctor, did they offer any type of treatment for the cognitive dysfunction? How did they approach that?

Terri: The approach was really to get me feeling better and understanding the role of pacing. When I feel better overall, my brain works better—my attention, memory, word finding are all better. When I don't feel well and I'm in a crash, it can make it almost impossible to find words or to even feel like I'm clearly articulating what I'm trying to say.

Yochai: So it was more about regulating the symptoms rather than fixing the problem.

Terri: ME is an inflammatory disease, so we put me on some anti-inflammatory meds. We also realized I have an immune deficiency. I had some treatments for that. I think the goal was to try to restore my body as much as possible in the hopes that the brain would start working because the foundational things were in place. I know that there are some medications that people are trying for their cognitive dysfunction, and I think it's an important conversation to have with health care providers. The ME/CFS Clinician Coalition website has a list of potentially helpful medications that people can bring to their provider.

When considering medications you may want to pursue, it's important to keep in mind that different approaches can be helpful for different people because people with Long COVID and ME/CFS have a range of severity and experiences in terms of their cognitive dysfunction.

I've personally been a little cautious about certain medications being helpful, like stimulants, but I really recommend having a conversation with your health care provider to see what works best.

I recognize that we're having our conversation right now about my experience with cognitive dysfunction, as it relates to the fact that I'm a person living with ME/CFS, but these issues I've faced are very similar to what people with Long COVID are experiencing. Although they're not perfectly aligned, I think a lot of the things that we experience really mirror one another.

Yochai: Absolutely, and the ME/CFS community has had decades of experience learning how to manage the symptoms and how to approach them. This is something that the Long COVID community can learn from them.

Terri: Exactly. Actually, I want to share some tips or tricks that have helped me. First, there are a lot of things around the role of technology. There's a pill that I have to take twice a day, and I so often can't remember it. I remember to take it at night because it's right next to my bed, but I can't remember to take it when I wake up. So, I've utilized phone alarms or a calendar—some technology to help me remember. Another thing that has helped me is writing things down—in a to-do list on a calendar or a sticky note.

Sometimes I've actually asked my family to help remind me about things, to organize things. I'm about to move out of my apartment, and I realized I'm just not going to be able to live my daily life and try to organize and think through the flow of a move, so I reached out to my mother and asked her to help me organize and remind me what I needed for a move. That was really helpful to preserve or conserve some of my brain energy.

Like I said before, my cognitive symptoms are worse when I overall don't feel well, so it's been helpful to think through ways that I can be as healthy as possible. Things like limiting how much my brain gets stimulated through music or sound or light or really anything that could require me to use brain energy.

So, it's really more thinking about crashes and post-exertional malaise—the key is understanding that when we talk about post-exertional malaise, we're also talking about physical, emotional, and mental exertion. For example, if you read a book or you watch a movie and then you crash the next day, your brain fog tends to be worse because you were overusing your brain. I think a lot of people might think about post-exertional malaise or crashes as only being related to physical exertion, like doing a load of laundry or cooking a meal. But it's not just physical; it can be cognitive effort, too.

If you're trying to tap into something to help you reach a clearer mind, maybe ask yourself a question about an activity you are about to engage in. For example, if you are about to watch a movie, do you need to watch it now or can you watch it later or in smaller pieces? Does that book need to be read in one sitting, or can you break it up into pieces? We refer to this practice in the ME/CFS community as *pacing* (see chapter 3).

Yochai: So, you've effectively found ways to navigate your life around the symptoms to try and avoid crashes to the best of your ability. But those crashes aren't fully predictable or fully avoidable. There are times when the disease rears its ugly head that are unpredictable and there's natural waxing and waning of the disease itself, right?

Terri: Yeah. I'm not perfect, and neither is my pacing. It's hard, because in the United States, there's this culture of work, work, work. You're only valued if you produce and so, whether you are conscious of that or not, we've all had this ingrained into our psyche somehow. It's this real push and pull of convincing yourself that you're a valuable person, even if you can't work in the way society expects of you.

If you got zero things checked off your list today, even if you may have had eight things on the list overall, that's okay. If you can only get one task done, maybe that's all you should strive for. And if you still don't get one item off your list that day, it's okay. We have to give ourselves some love to allow for some healing. We have to stop buying into some of these cultural narratives that we've all been taught—that you're not valuable or you're not the best person you could be.

I love the beauty of the "Stop. Rest. Pace." campaign of #MEAction (see chapter 3). It really is to the point. We know that pacing can help the body. It can help the mind. When I get into bed at a decent hour, when I don't try to be

Wonder Woman and do fourteen thousand things, I feel better the next day and my brain's clearer.

Yochai: And what you can or can't handle might be very different from someone else with the same diagnosis.

Terri: Absolutely. I think we all know health is on a continuum and people have different severities and breadth of their chronic disease and their cognitive dysfunction. I can only speak to what happens with my body, and it may be very different for somebody else. We really have to advocate for an individualized approach to our health care, and that includes what happens to us neurologically.

Yochai: Yeah. It sounds like the process of learning how to manage with this disease—and the cognitive symptoms specifically—is one of the first steps in getting to know this new version of yourself.

There's something that I think is crucial when thinking about "Stop. Rest. Pace." Even though you have some ability to control some of it, on the flip side, if someone thinks that they can exert full control over things, and then they have a crash, they can blame themselves for the crash. And I think that component of self-blame is particularly challenging, so it's important to recognize that even if you do give maximum effort to pace yourself appropriately, there will be some times that you crash and it isn't your fault.

Terri: Yeah, it's very important to not blame ourselves for our disease. We have so many other people around the world who want to blame us for our disease or misdiagnose us or say that it's a psychiatric illness when we know that it's not. The first year that I was diagnosed with ME/CFS, it was tough. I had to work toward eventually coming to a place of acceptance with this new identity. "Who was Terri before versus who is Terri now? And am I okay with who I am? Am I embarrassed by my brain and my body not working the way they used to? Do I want people in my family or my friends to know that this is part of who I am?"

I'm a person with a chronic disease. Really processing that, I experienced a lot of grief and anxiety that first year. *How long is this going to be? Is it forever?* I was still learning. I was shocked that there was no FDA-approved drug, that we don't have a biomarker. *How could this be? People have had this disease for decades.* I was thinking about what it would mean for me to be Terri with a disability, and allowing myself to grieve my healthy self. Then, coming to a place of *I'm still a valuable person with a chronic disease and a disability. I still have important things to contribute to the world.* But it was definitely a process, because I was pretty scared the first year of my diagnosis, entering this land that I wasn't familiar with and encountering this disease that nobody seemed to care about.

Yochai: Did you have people in your personal life who were really important to you in helping you manage the cognitive symptoms specifically?

Terri: Yeah. The one memory that I have that really resonated with me about this is a really good friend. I was talking to my friend, Olivia, on the phone and, all of a sudden, I couldn't remember what we were talking about. I just literally stopped talking, and I started to tear up, saying "I cannot remember what we're talking about. I don't know what word I'm trying to find in my brain."

She was just so supportive and kind and said, "It's okay, take your time. We can change the subject, and we can talk about something else." She reminded me of what we were talking about. I just remember her kindness and her love and her patience. She didn't make me feel embarrassed or feel any discomfort. I think this is probably one of the most lovely memories I have of anybody in my life, and it really meant a lot. I've never forgotten that she did that.

Yochai: We all need more people like that in our lives.

Terri: Everybody needs an Olivia in their lives.

Yochai: I colead a Long COVID supportive psychotherapy group, and several of the people in the group have cognitive dysfunction/brain fog. It's clear that having someone who can help these people manage the things that are challenging for them can be especially helpful. Somebody who can organize your doctor's appointments for you or some of the chores around the house.

Terri: When you're working with your clients, do you ever refer them for neuropsychological testing? What are some of the things that you think about in terms of services or support that might be helpful, especially for people who are really struggling with cognitive dysfunction?

Yochai: I treat people for psychiatric or psychological challenges that come along with Long COVID, so often I'm referring them to another provider, like a neurologist, who will specifically address the cognitive dysfunction. They sometimes will do neuropsychological testing as a way to get a better sense of what the person's cognitive issues specifically are. They can look at things like memory, motor functioning, verbal functioning, fluency, and then more generally your ability to learn, think, understand, and problem-solve, executive functioning.

These are all things that you touched on in talking about how your cognitive symptoms have influenced your ability to interact with the world, and neuropsychological testing will specifically look at all of those things. One of the challenges, though, is that many people don't have information about what their baseline cognitive functioning used to be, so it can be hard to really assess the changes that may have occurred once the disease presents itself. Nonetheless, this sort of testing can be helpful for some people, and if there are gross abnormalities, that information might be helpful for insurance companies if you're applying for disability.

Another thing that some people are looking at in the research side of things is quantitative electroencephalography (qEEG), a way to visualize electrical activity in the brain. The neuropsych testing basically shows you the ways in which you're not functioning well, and then the quantitative EEG can show you where in the brain you're not functioning well.

So those are diagnostic tools that can be helpful, and then in terms of treatment, the only thing that I'm aware of that people are doing (other than some medication trials) is cognitive rehab, which allows people to do exercises that are specifically targeted to address the areas in which they're struggling and hopefully, over time, to learn ways to cope with that dysfunction or to relearn some of those things. That can be quite helpful and also very challenging.

Terri: So when you use the word *exercise* around cognitive rehab, what would be an example of an exercise that might be assigned to a person?

Yochai: There're all sorts of memory tests and exercises, depending on the type of memory issues the person is having. It depends on the program and what the nature of the dysfunction is. It ranges from simple stuff, like relearning how to brush your teeth, to more complicated, complex tasks.

Terri: Yeah, that sounds like it could be really helpful for people. I shared earlier that when you have cognitive dysfunction, it can impact your ability to do paid work. People may have some fear around this. I'd advise talking to human resources about work accommodations just to see what the policies are and what is legally available to you. Find out if there's flexibility in the hours or the tasks that you do. There are some people who may have to consider leaving work because of disability, and that's going to be a really difficult decision to make.

How do you make that decision? How do you decide when you may need to leave work? I think you start thinking about it when you start noticing significant changes in how you work and how much work you're able to do. It's certainly worth considering if you get to a point where work just isn't sustainable for you anymore. You may realize, *I don't think I can do this anymore—I need to start finding out about the process of leaving work.*

It's a process to get disability; it requires a lot of documentation. It also requires a lot of conversations, not only with your boss, but also with your family or your loved ones. It's probably a good idea to have a friend or a family member or a buddy to help you navigate that process. Institutions don't make it easy for people to navigate systems, and it can be overwhelming, especially if you're already having difficulty around cognitive issues. And if you're having cognitive difficulties, how do you stay organized? How do you process all the steps? Having somebody who can partner with you to navigate that together will hopefully make it less confusing so you can get approved for the services that you definitely need. There are people who've been successful getting approved for disability benefits, but there can also be many disappointments and challenges in the process.

Yochai: The truth is that insurance companies don't make it easy for anyone to navigate these systems. If you have cognitive dysfunction, I can imagine it might feel impossible sometimes.

Terri: Exactly. I'm aware there are some concerns about individuals who might try to feign disability to game the system, but I've honestly never met a person with ME/CFS or with Long COVID who hasn't wanted their job, who hasn't wanted back their pre-COVID, pre-ME/CFS life. I have never, ever heard anybody say, "Oh, I don't want to work. I don't want my life the way it was before." People want their lives back.

Yochai: Yeah. In fact, often people overcommit and try to cling to their prior life, even if it does cause many crashes, because it's so challenging to let go of that.

It can also be helpful to modify your work hours, if your workplace will allow. Because this disease can be somewhat unpredictable, having some flexibility in the form of a set number of hours a week that you can use at whatever time you like, for example, can be helpful. A job like that can allow for the gratification of continuing to work and help prevent you from pushing yourself too hard.

Terri: Yeah. I think those are important conversations to have with human resources—not only about hours, but maybe you can change jobs. Maybe the tasks that you do need to change.

I'm so glad we're having this conversation. I know you are part of the Patient-Led Research Collaborative, and one of the things that was captured in your survey of people with Long COVID was that 88 percent of the total respondents, which was 3,310 at the time, experienced cognitive dysfunction or memory loss, at similar rates across all age groups.

So, this is really a key symptom that people are reporting, and I'm really hoping that science and research is going to be expedited to really help people in this area.

Going back to the beauty of groups, places like Body Politic, #MEAction, and Long COVID Facebook pages help people stay on top of developments in science and medicine so that they can have early access as soon as there are some really concrete interventions that are proven to help people.

Yochai: Absolutely, and there are some pretty motivated, smart minds out there who are really working on this issue. Just recently there was a paper out, looking at changes within the brain that come after COVID. I imagine that now there'll be an attempt to correlate those to neuropsychological changes, and I'm optimistic for what the future holds in terms of addressing this problem.

You touched on how common cognitive dysfunction is in Long COVID, and the other important thing to mention is that its presentation is often delayed. The average onset of cognitive dysfunction in our cohort peaked around three months after COVID symptoms first started. So, it's important to recognize that it's something that can be delayed and sometimes it might get missed because of that.

Terri: Yeah, exactly. I have a friend who is having a lot of challenges around Long COVID, and you have these symptoms at onset and then something comes three months later, or six months later, nine months later. You're just thinking,

Is a new symptom coming every quarter? Since 2016, I'm more conscious of my body and my health, and I take extra care when going to medical appointments to try to be the best narrator I can be. I also started recording my medical appointments so that I can listen to them later in case I miss something, or if I just can't quite grasp what is being said at that moment if I'm not having the best cognitive day. Those kinds of things can help. I try to stay true to the fact that I'm the best assessor of my body. Sometimes it helps to have someone else come with me, too. That way they can pay attention to what's being said and help me communicate my needs if I'm unable to in the moment.

Yochai: Absolutely. Well, thank you very much for taking the time and for sharing some of your personal experiences. I know it's not always easy.

Terri: Thanks for having a conversation with me today, too. I think that we all have to come from a place of community collaboration and health justice in everything that we do, because we're all connected, and that's become more and more real through the COVID pandemic. We have to take care of one another, and we have to love one another. That's why I felt safe sharing my story today. I don't want other people to go through this, and hopefully everything we talked about today will help people.

Survival Tips

- Life Tips
  - » Consider workplace accommodations: Terri worked with her editor to find a way to continue publishing journalistic work via transcribed interviews, even when cognitive symptoms made it difficult to write.
  - » Rely on family and friends: Ask for support when you need it, and consider bringing a loved one with you to your health care provider's appointments.
  - » Seek support from others: People with chronic diseases often do better when they can talk to another person about it. It can be even better if it's a person who is going through the same experience. Some resources available to people to gain support around their cognitive dysfunction include the following:

- #MEAction's Long Covid Facebook Group
- Body Politic: This site is organized with specific Slack channels to connect and share information.
- Bateman Horne Center: They have a guidebook for people with ME/CFS that has tips for managing/navigating cognitive difficulties.
- Medical professionals: Your provider should be supportive of you and help you brainstorm. They should be willing to consider drugs used in other diseases as detailed in the ME/CFS Clinician Coalition treatment recommendations, and they should keep up with what's happening in the field of science and research.

» Don't make big decisions on a bad day: If you're not understanding information, receiving information the way it's intended, or even being able to verbally communicate or write, it's probably not the best day to make a big decision on something that's important.

• Health Care Tips

» Record appointments with health care providers: With your provider's permission, it may be helpful to take audio recordings of your health care appointments so you don't have to recall all the details from memory, or take notes while dealing with brain fog.

» Track symptoms over time: Remember that cognitive dysfunction can sometimes be a delayed Long COVID symptom. This means you may not notice the impacts immediately after your initial infection. Keep track of how symptoms wax and wane over time to learn more about yourself.

» Consider multiple approaches: Often, managing cognitive dysfunction is more about regulating the symptoms than fixing the problem. You may consider pursuing medications, lifestyle changes, memory retraining tests and exercises, or other tests that can measure function. Symptoms vary and there is a spectrum of severity, so there is no one-size-fits-all approach.

» Consider using pillboxes: Since you may be trying lots of different medications or supplements for different things that are going on with your body, pillboxes can be helpful for organizing so that you don't forget or get confused about what pills you took.

- Pacing Tips

  » Pace yourself: Break up large or complicated energy-draining activities into smaller bite-sized tasks, and schedule planned rest in between. This goes for TV and movies as well! You may find it's better to break them up into smaller chunks.

  » Cut yourself some slack: No one is perfect at pacing or managing their cognitive symptoms. Some days will be harder than others. The widespread culture of productivity in our society may sometimes make you feel like you're not worthy. As much as possible, push back on these cultural narratives. You are valuable and important, regardless of your productivity.

  » Limit your time on social media: Track how much time online feels like too much time and consider setting timers to remind yourself to log off, so you don't become too overwhelmed or trigger a crash.

  » Consider communication cards: If you're a person who's more severely ill or having a really bad day, and you just cannot put together a sentence or it's hard to kind of think through how to communicate what you want, you can ask a family member or friend to ask you yes or no questions and then you can have a communication card that says yes or no.

  » Utilize technology: Set reminders on your phone or computer to help manage daily tasks. Using a digital calendar with built in reminders may help. Regular old sticky notes may work, too!

  » Consider limiting Zoom sessions: Although Zoom can provide us with sometimes much-needed social time, it can also be exhausting. We recommend setting a limit for Zoom calls. For example, if you know you can't stay on a call for more than thirty minutes, consider setting a timer and/or communicating clear time boundaries with whoever you are Zooming with.

  » Use voice memo messaging: Smartphones have a voice memo function, where you can click a little microphone and say what you need to say, and it'll type it out for you, or it will record it with an option to send to the receiver as text. That can be a great way to conserve some energy.

CHAPTER 9

NOT THE ONLY ONE
TALKING ABOUT MENSTRUAL CHANGES

Monique Jackson

I EXPERIENCED CHANGES TO MY MENSTRUAL CYCLE AFTER
FALLING ILL FROM A SUSPECTED INFECTION OF COVID-19. UNTIL
NOW, I HAVE STRUGGLED TO IDENTIFY AND ARTICULATE MY
EXPERIENCES.

 I REACHED OUT TO OTHERS WHO HAD ALSO NOTICED
CHANGES, TO SHARE AND REFLECT ON WHAT WE THINK AND
FEEL IS HAPPENING IN OUR BODIES. THE CONVERSATIONS
BELOW ARE BASED ON TRANSCRIPTS OF RECORDINGS OR CHATS
EXCHANGED WITH OTHER LONG-HAULERS ONLINE. THEY HAVE
BEEN EDITED SLIGHTLY FOR BREVITY AND CLARITY.

PEOPLE INVOLVED

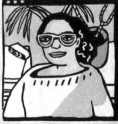

MONIQUE JACKSON
SHE/HER
33 YEARS OLD
BIRACIAL
ENGLISH, AMERICAN
LONDON, UK
DATE OF INFECTION:
MARCH 2020

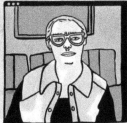

BORIS GAY
THEY/THEM
34 YEARS OLD
WHITE
SCOTTISH
GLASGOW, SCOTLAND
DATE OF INFECTION:
JANUARY 2021

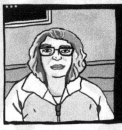

JO DAINOW
SHE/HER
56 YEARS OLD
WHITE
ENGLISH
LONDON, UK
DATE OF INFECTION:
MARCH 2020

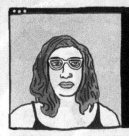

LETÍCIA SOARES
SHE/HER
37 YEARS OLD
BIRACIAL
BRAZILIAN
BRAZIL
DATE OF INFECTION:
APRIL 2020

BORIS & MONIQUE   MARCH 8, 2022

I met Boris Gay via a callout on my social media. I wanted to speak with a nonbinary person who had experienced Long COVID–related menstrual changes in order to compare experiences and gain insight into perspectives other than my own.

Boris was candid about their difficulties navigating the health care system in Scotland. While it's still a part of the United Kingdom's National Health Service, Scotland's health care system has some distinct differences in opportunities to access medical care, compared to what I experienced in London, England.

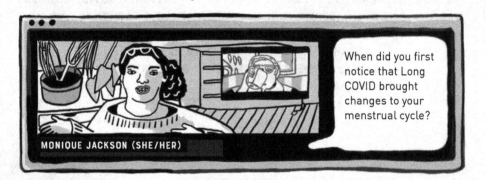

MONIQUE JACKSON (SHE/HER)

When did you first notice that Long COVID brought changes to your menstrual cycle?

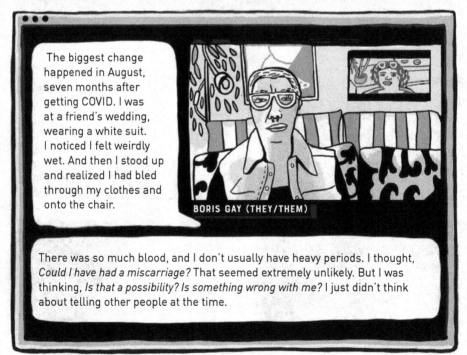

The biggest change happened in August, seven months after getting COVID. I was at a friend's wedding, wearing a white suit. I noticed I felt weirdly wet. And then I stood up and realized I had bled through my clothes and onto the chair.

BORIS GAY (THEY/THEM)

There was so much blood, and I don't usually have heavy periods. I thought, *Could I have had a miscarriage?* That seemed extremely unlikely. But I was thinking, *Is that a possibility? Is something wrong with me?* I just didn't think about telling other people at the time.

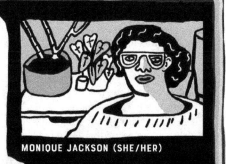

That is scary. I'm sorry you went through that. I relate to feeling unsure of what changes are going on as a result of COVID. I'm thirty-three; I've been menstruating for a long time. And, yet, it's hard to know in what way my hormones or periods have changed since COVID and how to talk to others about it.

MONIQUE JACKSON (SHE/HER)

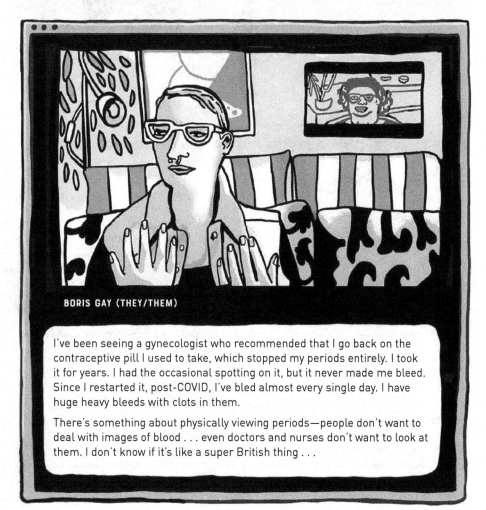

BORIS GAY (THEY/THEM)

I've been seeing a gynecologist who recommended that I go back on the contraceptive pill I used to take, which stopped my periods entirely. I took it for years. I had the occasional spotting on it, but it never made me bleed. Since I restarted it, post-COVID, I've bled almost every single day. I have huge heavy bleeds with clots in them.

There's something about physically viewing periods—people don't want to deal with images of blood . . . even doctors and nurses don't want to look at them. I don't know if it's like a super British thing . . .

BORIS GAY (THEY/THEM)

I've been taking photos of clots. I ended up sending them to a friend of mine saying, "I hope you don't mind me sending this to you, but what's your take on this?" They're also a non-binary friend who has had bad problems with periods. They were like, "I've had clots like that before. But if it's not normal for you, you should keep telling people about this."

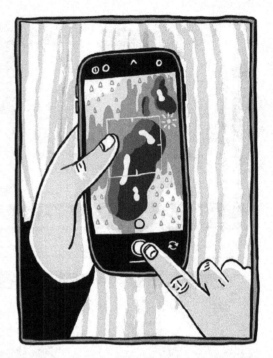

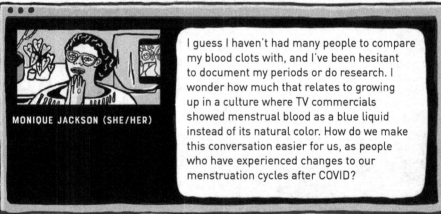

MONIQUE JACKSON (SHE/HER)

I guess I haven't had many people to compare my blood clots with, and I've been hesitant to document my periods or do research. I wonder how much that relates to growing up in a culture where TV commercials showed menstrual blood as a blue liquid instead of its natural color. How do we make this conversation easier for us, as people who have experienced changes to our menstruation cycles after COVID?

BORIS GAY (THEY/THEM)

That's hard. I guess we just all need to keep talking about it in public places. If social media didn't exist, I keep thinking, if the pandemic had happened even a decade ago, how lonely it would have been, and how hard it would have been to be in contact with other people who share these experiences. I'm extremely grateful to talk to you and to have somebody. Just listening to you and the way you're responding to me, I feel like somebody is taking what I'm saying seriously, and I really appreciate that. It feels nice to have somebody say, "You're not alone in this."

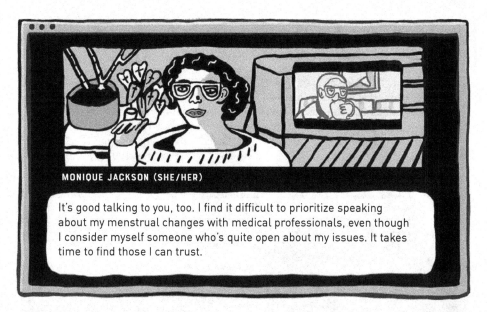

MONIQUE JACKSON (SHE/HER)

It's good talking to you, too. I find it difficult to prioritize speaking about my menstrual changes with medical professionals, even though I consider myself someone who's quite open about my issues. It takes time to find those I can trust.

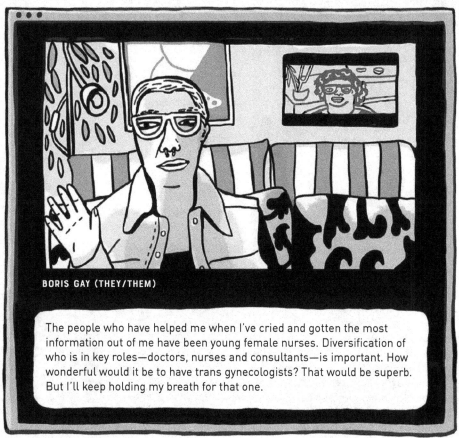

BORIS GAY (THEY/THEM)

The people who have helped me when I've cried and gotten the most information out of me have been young female nurses. Diversification of who is in key roles—doctors, nurses and consultants—is important. How wonderful would it be to have trans gynecologists? That would be superb. But I'll keep holding my breath for that one.

LETÍCIA & MONIQUE   MARCH 8, 2022

Letícia and I started messaging each other online in October 2020 after finding and commenting on each other's various Long COVID advocacy posts on social media. It must have been through Long COVID community pages that we first made contact, as we had no mutual friends and live in different countries. I wanted to get Letícia's perspective, in part because she migrated during the pandemic between Canada and Brazil, and I hoped to compare our experiences of private and nationalized medical care.

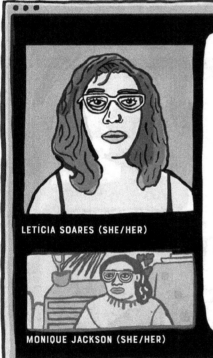

LETÍCIA SOARES (SHE/HER)

MONIQUE JACKSON (SHE/HER)

I've had my Mirena IUD since 2012. Most of the time, I didn't have a period at all. When I got COVID and then Long COVID, I was sick for so long and having so many crashes all the time, so it's very hard to pinpoint whether there were menstrual cycle changes. I always heard people in our support group talk about it, and I'd be like, shit, maybe my crashes are related to my menstrual cycle . . . but I have no way of knowing that because of my IUD.

The very worst experience that I had was when I got my first period after being infected with COVID—my first period in years. I woke up suddenly in the middle of the night, feeling like I couldn't breathe, and opened all the windows. I felt so hot, like a human

LETÍCIA SOARES (SHE/HER)

torch. Then, a month or two later during my next menstrual cycle, I woke up in the middle of the night again. I looked at my phone—it was 3:39 AM—and I just started crying. My body woke me up to have intrusive thoughts and just cry my ass off. It is so, so strange. I think I now have a sleep pattern disturbance in general. I'm now on sleep medication.

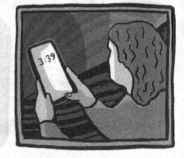

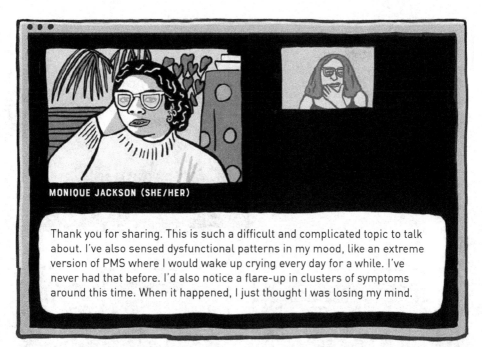

MONIQUE JACKSON (SHE/HER)

Thank you for sharing. This is such a difficult and complicated topic to talk about. I've also sensed dysfunctional patterns in my mood, like an extreme version of PMS where I would wake up crying every day for a while. I've never had that before. I'd also notice a flare-up in clusters of symptoms around this time. When it happened, I just thought I was losing my mind.

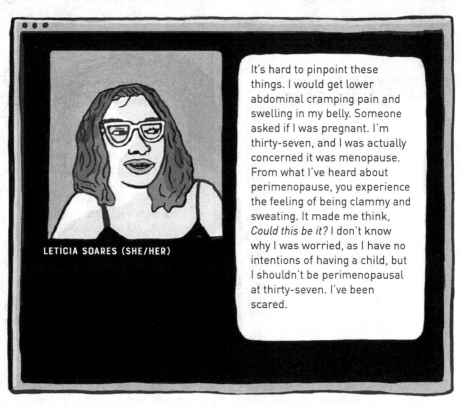

LETÍCIA SOARES (SHE/HER)

It's hard to pinpoint these things. I would get lower abdominal cramping pain and swelling in my belly. Someone asked if I was pregnant. I'm thirty-seven, and I was actually concerned it was menopause. From what I've heard about perimenopause, you experience the feeling of being clammy and sweating. It made me think, *Could this be it?* I don't know why I was worried, as I have no intentions of having a child, but I shouldn't be perimenopausal at thirty-seven. I've been scared.

LETÍCIA SOARES (SHE/HER)

I feel like we understate the physiological processes that go on in our bodies that translate into mental health symptoms. I am grateful, though, that I can express these feelings with my partner. They help me shower every day and get out of the house.

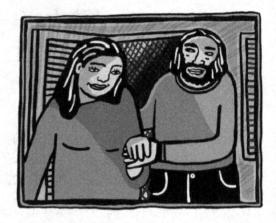

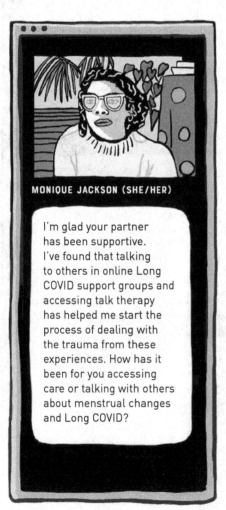

MONIQUE JACKSON (SHE/HER)

I'm glad your partner has been supportive. I've found that talking to others in online Long COVID support groups and accessing talk therapy has helped me start the process of dealing with the trauma from these experiences. How has it been for you accessing care or talking with others about menstrual changes and Long COVID?

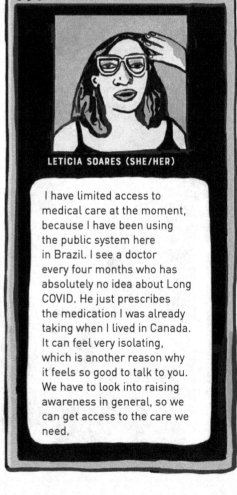

LETÍCIA SOARES (SHE/HER)

I have limited access to medical care at the moment, because I have been using the public system here in Brazil. I see a doctor every four months who has absolutely no idea about Long COVID. He just prescribes the medication I was already taking when I lived in Canada. It can feel very isolating, which is another reason why it feels so good to talk to you. We have to look into raising awareness in general, so we can get access to the care we need.

JO & MONIQUE

MARCH 8, 2022

Jo and I met through our work on Long Covid Support, an international peer support group. I appreciate Jo speaking about her experiences with menopause and the relationship between aging and Long COVID. It was helpful to talk with each other and share intergenerational knowledge about the changes we noticed in our mood and well-being.

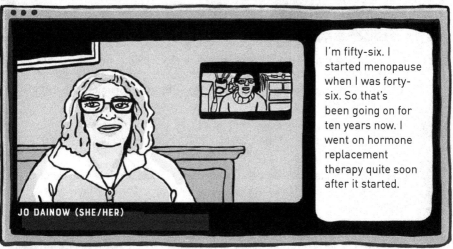

I'm fifty-six. I started menopause when I was forty-six. So that's been going on for ten years now. I went on hormone replacement therapy quite soon after it started.

JO DAINOW (SHE/HER)

JO DAINOW (SHE/HER)

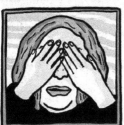

Ten years ago, I was really . . . exhausted. I was shaking all the time and had brain fog. It made me feel really rough, to the point that I wasn't able to go into work. I used to crawl around at home because I just didn't have the energy to do anything.

I thought it was a virus. After a while, I realized it happened in cycles. For two weeks, I was fine, but the following two weeks, I wasn't fine. So, I went on estrogen, and it made a massive difference.

I got COVID back in March 2020. I had it for two weeks, and then felt better. But by that point, we were in lockdown. I started to feel sick again. It was very similar to how I felt when I thought I'd had a virus before but was actually going through perimenopause.

A couple of months after I had COVID, I noticed my periods were coming in fits and starts and doing really weird things. I was having quite a lot of pelvic pain. But I didn't think anything of it, because I'm older and had dealt with menopause. I thought, *Well, maybe this is just me changing.*

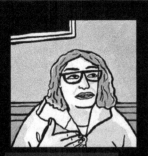

JO DAINOW (SHE/HER)

In June and July of 2020, my periods were so much worse than I had ever experienced before. It was painful from ovulation to mid-cycle, right through to when I had my period, and my period was coming early. My cycle was erratic: In one cycle, my period would come after twenty-one days; the next, it might come after twenty-eight, and then back to twenty-one. It was really all over the place. And in the time around my period, I also noticed the worsening of my Long COVID symptoms in general. As soon as I was mid-cycle, I would notice a real increase in fatigue and cognitive issues. I get a bit of nausea now, too, before my period starts.

There were other changes, too, that took place after I was infected with COVID: I gained weight. My hair became really horrible and brittle. My skin became quite puffy.

I still have irregular periods, pain, headaches, fatigue, and brain fog. And now I'm at the point where I don't really know what is hormonal and what's Long COVID.

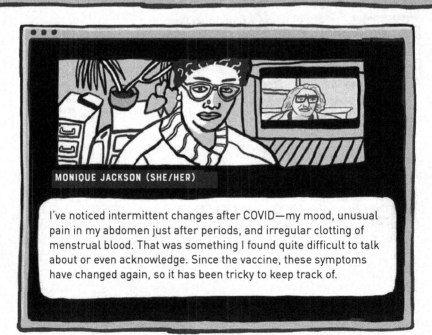

MONIQUE JACKSON (SHE/HER)

I've noticed intermittent changes after COVID—my mood, unusual pain in my abdomen just after periods, and irregular clotting of menstrual blood. That was something I found quite difficult to talk about or even acknowledge. Since the vaccine, these symptoms have changed again, so it has been tricky to keep track of.

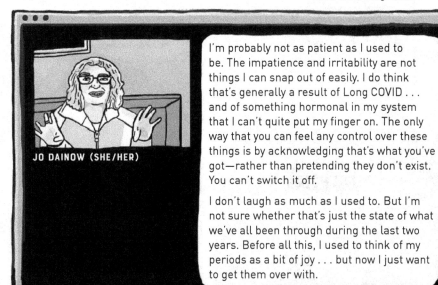

JO DAINOW (SHE/HER)

I'm probably not as patient as I used to be. The impatience and irritability are not things I can snap out of easily. I do think that's generally a result of Long COVID . . . and of something hormonal in my system that I can't quite put my finger on. The only way that you can feel any control over these things is by acknowledging that's what you've got—rather than pretending they don't exist. You can't switch it off.

I don't laugh as much as I used to. But I'm not sure whether that's just the state of what we've all been through during the last two years. Before all this, I used to think of my periods as a bit of joy . . . but now I just want to get them over with.

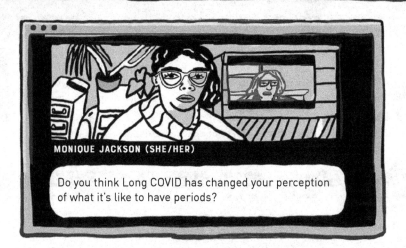

MONIQUE JACKSON (SHE/HER)

Do you think Long COVID has changed your perception of what it's like to have periods?

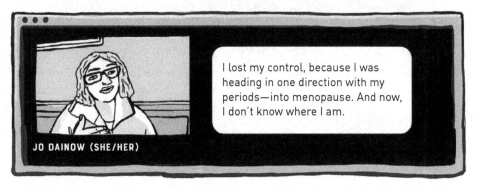

JO DAINOW (SHE/HER)

I lost my control, because I was heading in one direction with my periods—into menopause. And now, I don't know where I am.

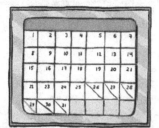

JO DAINOW (SHE/HER)

I used to work with a whole load of women and we all used to sync up, you know, they say you synchronize your periods.

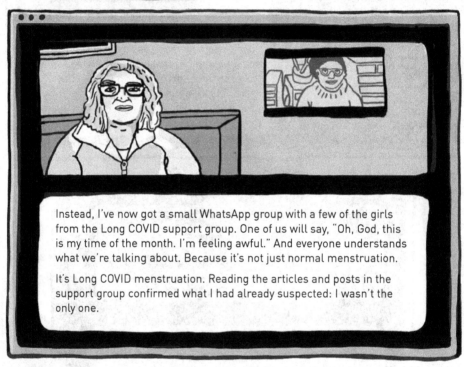

Instead, I've now got a small WhatsApp group with a few of the girls from the Long COVID support group. One of us will say, "Oh, God, this is my time of the month. I'm feeling awful." And everyone understands what we're talking about. Because it's not just normal menstruation.

It's Long COVID menstruation. Reading the articles and posts in the support group confirmed what I had already suspected: I wasn't the only one.

These series of online conversations about menstrual changes brought on by Long COVID have been simultaneously insightful and difficult for me to have. It's been a real privilege to be able to connect with others about a subject that I have struggled to recognize in myself. Thanks to Boris, Jo, and Letícia for trusting me to re-share our conversations about what we are feeling in our bodies. It's my hope that, by sharing these conversations, we will help others feel less alone.

SURVIVAL TIPS

1. Understand that your period may change as a result of Long COVID—if you are experiencing unusual periods, worsened Long COVID symptoms during your period, or new difficulties with temperature regulation and migraines during your menstrual cycle, among other issues, you may be experiencing Long COVID periods.

2. Document changes to your periods and mood alongside other changes that may have occurred after a COVID-19 infection. Track your symptoms around your cycle.

3. Talk about what you're experiencing with supportive people you trust. Start with whoever you feel least embarrassed to talk to. This might be a friend or loved one, or it could be a stranger on the internet!

4. Find peer-advice in Long COVID support groups. Look out for posts about new research on COVID and menstrual periods or COVID and hormones.

5. Seek out diverse health care providers or health care providers with personal experience of menstruation.

6. If you are experiencing intense mental health issues during or near your menstrual periods, consider educating yourself on premenstrual dysphoric disorder (PMDD) and seeking out gynecologists and mental health professionals with experience in PMDD.

CHAPTER 10

The Search for Community

Finding Peer-to-Peer Support

Padma Priya DVL

I t started as a bad headache; like really bad. I experience chronic migraines, but the intensity of this headache was like nothing I'd ever felt before. I had been reporting on the unfolding coronavirus for two months—so I was immediately concerned. Then came the overwhelming feeling of exhaustion, similar to what I've felt before when a fever is about to set in.

It was April 2020, amidst India's harshest lockdown, that my health, and with it my life, began to unravel. As a journalist and cofounder of Suno India, a podcast-only digital media platform, my team and I had begun covering COVID in February 2020. We were investigating India's readiness to handle the pandemic, considering our underdeveloped public health care infrastructure, among many other factors. Then, a pandemic-induced migrant exodus began and we saw a humanitarian crisis unfold as millions of people were displaced by a national lockdown that was announced with just one day's notice. This meant millions of people, mostly working-class, began an arduous journey back to their respective hometowns—many on foot, walking hundreds of miles. An estimated 40 million people were affected.[1] While the team and I were forced to switch to reporting using digital tools, other aspects of our day-to-day lives were affected, too. It was during this time, I suspect (as I may never truly know), on one of our visits to stock up on supplies, that the virus came calling for me.

As soon as the headache arrived, I immediately isolated myself, even though my family members felt I was being a tad paranoid. On day two, I developed a 100°F (38°C) fever, which soon increased to 102°F (39°C). I knew it was bad because it was accompanied by chills, bone pain, and terrible night sweats. On day three, I called the government helpline to get a test and was told to go to a tertiary government hospital in Hyderabad, the city where I live. No ambulances were available. My husband, Rakesh, had to drive me to the hospital with our then-four-year-old in tow. The fear we both had in our hearts was primal; even just being dropped off for the test was emotionally draining. After waiting for a few hours, I was turned away, denied a test because I was "young enough" (I was almost thirty-four years old) and my symptoms "didn't seem as severe as some other patients." I had a high fever and a dry cough, which would worsen as the days went by. I watched as another woman, seven months pregnant, was also turned away for similar reasons. We were both sent home to manage our care alone, given only Tylenol and Zithromax and no advice about what to do if our symptoms worsened.

At this time, the Indian government was disallowing private hospitals and diagnostic centers from offering care or tests. Instead, they urged patients to pursue care at government hospitals, which they claimed were well-equipped. But my visit made clear that these health care systems were overwhelmed, and difficult decisions were being made about who to treat—and who to send home.

On day four, my breathing began to get labored. Out of sheer frustration (and because I'm a journalist), I felt the need to chronicle what I had experienced. So, I turned to Twitter, sharing a thread about my experience of developing symptoms and being denied care and testing.[2] The thread quickly went viral and was picked up by various media outlets, who reported on my attempt to get care and the low testing capacity in my area. It was only on day six, after my viral tweets, that I was called back to the hospital, admitted, and finally administered a test. The health care workers there performed X-rays and a high-resolution CT scan of my lungs, but I never got to see my results. In fact, I was discharged quickly as my COVID-19 PCR test was negative, and the hospital where I'd sought care was designated for COVID care only. The health care workers treating me believed I didn't have COVID.

However, I was told I could pursue care at another hospital that wasn't only treating COVID patients. When I went there the next day, the doctors reviewed my reports from the previous day and took another X-ray of my chest. I received a clinical diagnosis of COVID-19, based on my symptoms, and yet I wasn't asked to return to the designated COVID hospital. Instead, they advised me to isolate at home.

A week had passed since my symptoms first began; I was experiencing severe drops in my oxygen levels throughout the day. My dry cough had also worsened, and I now felt breathless. I was advised to isolate for twenty-one days—a far cry from our current shorter and riskier recommendations! I stayed in my bedroom for all three weeks and sent my child to my parents' house. Rakesh stayed with me to care for me, ensure I ate well, and do his best to keep up my spirits, but he had to isolate himself in another room to avoid infection. The isolation was nerve-wracking, and no amount of streaming services or books helped. I missed my family and my child, and I desperately wanted a hug. A dear friend who was a pulmonologist at a COVID hospital ward in Mumbai checked on me via video consultations and advised me over the course of those three weeks.

It was during one of those nights, while scrolling Facebook, that I came across a support group for COVID patients and survivors. Later on, I would discover others. The conversations people were having in these groups, while sometimes alarming, mostly helped me stay grounded. The advice patients were giving one another to cope with this novel deadly virus was calming. Finally, I had found others like me who were in isolation or had gone through isolation and understood how lonely that experience can be. Some had coped better than others. I didn't cope well, but finally having the support of others helped.

I must also mention the role that my friends played during this time, forming a sort of support group of their own. Some of them checked in on me multiple times a day. My best friend Krishna, who lives in Australia, was a lifesaver during many nights when I was wrecked by the fever and couldn't sleep. She would help to distract me from my physical pain by sending me beautiful pictures of bright blue skies or talking about our time together in high school.

By mid-May 2020, I was out of isolation and welcomed my thirty-fourth year with my family. By June, I was back to working at my company and reporting on the COVID pandemic. But all the while, I continued to experience the aftereffects of my COVID infection. I would become breathless doing simple, previously joyful things, like picking my daughter up or taking a short walk down the street. My insomnia was intolerable and no amount of mindfulness activities or cutting down on caffeine helped me sleep. I continued to have bizarre dreams, which had begun with my initial infection. Only later, in the support groups, did I read that many people were experiencing these vivid, lifelike "COVID nightmares."

Each time I noticed a new symptom, my immediate response was doubt. I don't know if it was because I didn't want to be sick or because the news and public health guidelines didn't acknowledge any of my symptoms, but I began to gaslight myself. I told myself that it was probably exhaustion and that my body was still recovering. I figured my anxiety was turning me into a hypochondriac; earlier in life, I had been gaslit by doctors who accused me of "faking" an illness, which left me with lingering emotional scars and worries that maybe I was just imagining it all. But a little part of me, almost instinctively, knew that something was "off" about my body.

At this point, little was known about Long COVID in India and there was very little help or explanation from public health authorities as to what could be happening. My pulmonologist friend, Dr. Sarthak, speculated that my ongoing symptoms were probably a part of a post-viral illness. Later, I would learn that post-viral illnesses aren't new in India; in fact, they're quite common. Dengue and chikungunya, two viruses spread to humans from mosquitoes, are endemic here, and I eventually learned that many people with these infections also go on to develop chronic health issues.[3]

Eventually, when new symptoms popped up and I found myself questioning everything, I learned to check support groups to see if anyone else was experiencing the same thing. Finding these people was always a bittersweet moment because I didn't want anyone to be sick like me. At the same time, these interactions validated my gut instinct that I wasn't losing it and that there was something going wrong in my body.

Then, in July, the "crash" happened. I call it the "crash" because, since that day, my life has never been the same. A simple trip back from the grocers left me exhausted; I suddenly began sweating and felt my heart rate increase. Before I knew it, I had passed out near my apartment's elevator. Fear of COVID was so intense at that time that no one offered to even help me up, and I had to wait until Rakesh could come and get me. I rushed to my primary care doctor, who checked my vitals and found my heart rate elevated and my blood pressure very low. He advised rest, asked me to eat well, and said it was probably a onetime thing. It was not a onetime thing.

Over the next few weeks, I experienced many such attacks, which I learned were considered *syncopes*, but my doctors didn't provide much explanation of what this meant or how to manage it. Once again, I turned to my support groups and saw there were others like me experiencing similar symptoms. This was also the first time that I read the word *dysautonomia* (see chapter 2), and I was surprised to find that so many of my symptoms were similar to the ones that people with dysautonomia were describing. As the syncope attacks continued, I continued searching for answers. I reached out to a cardiologist who ran some tests, but the results were considered normal. I was told there was mild inflammation around my heart muscle but that this was not usual after a prolonged viral infection. My cardiologist said I was probably anxious and advised me to seek psychiatric help and prescribed supplements. A roadblock yet again!

I know what anxiety feels like, and I knew deep down that this was not anxiety. I went back to the support groups for help. Someone suggested I ask the cardiologist to run a Holter monitor test, which is essentially a twenty-four-hour electrocardiogram (ECG) that monitors one's heart rate by measuring the time between each beat. It is considered an accurate way of picking up on instances of bradycardia (slow heart rate) or tachycardia (fast heart rate).

I hadn't heard of this diagnostic tool, and I was excited to return to the cardiologist, armed with this new information. I told her that many others who were recovering from COVID-19 were experiencing similar symptoms and asked her to run additional tests including a Holter test. After much self-advocating on my part, she reluctantly prescribed the test. The results showed some abnormalities: There were 163 instances in which my heart rate was elevated for no evident reason. The cardiologist again suggested that my issue might be psychological, though she recommended that I increase the salt in my diet. I left that appointment feeling dejected, angry, and alone. I was angry because I could sense that, despite the Holter test results, she truly didn't believe there was anything "majorly wrong"— the exact words she used during our interaction.

I tried sprinkling more salt onto my food but saw little improvement. I know now—after attending a virtual conference on dysautonomia—that increased sodium intake can help some people with dysautonomia manage symptoms, but my cardiologist hadn't explained how much salt to add to my food or any other symptom-management techniques, and so the fatigue, brain fog, and fainting attacks continued.

As my physical health declined, so did my mental health. Again, it was the support groups that kept me going. I remember one particular night, when I was feeling intensely lonely and despairing, I went on Facebook and scrolled for hours, reading through others' experiences to help me ground myself. The support groups had become my lifeline, helping me to realize that I wasn't alone or "making it all up." I started therapy, because my illness journey was causing me anxiety, and I was soon diagnosed with clinical depression. My therapist recommended that I seek a psychiatrist's opinion and get a prescription for antidepressants. So, there I was, in September of 2020, five months from my original infection, physically and mentally exhausted, and making more progress on my mental health than my debilitating physical symptoms. But that was also the month that I finally caught a break.

Through another sort of support group—my virtual network of health journalists—I got in touch with a doctor who was treating people experiencing post-COVID symptoms. He put me in touch with an internist in my city. The internist, Dr. Guruprasad, heard me out, looked at all my existing reports, and then recommended I get some tests to check my norepinephrine, epinephrine, and cortisol levels, among other metrics of health. When the results came back, they showed highly elevated levels of norepinephrine and epinephrine—levels so high that Dr. Guruprasad told me they're usually only seen in athletes on performance-enhancing drugs.

He explained that there could only be a few reasons for my high levels. The first possibility was that I had an adrenal gland tumor. The other was that my autonomic nervous system, which is in charge of our blood pressure, heart rate, digestion, and other unconscious bodily processes, was malfunctioning by being stuck in fight-or-flight mode. I was relieved to discover—after spending another nerve-wracking week waiting for results—that I did not have a tumor. So, Dr. Guruprasad prescribed calcium blockers and anti-anxiety medicines (since heightened adrenaline levels can cause panic attacks and vice versa). The calcium blockers, he told me, would help with stabilizing my heart rate and adrenaline levels. The anti-anxiety medicines would help with my anxiety attacks. He also prescribed medicine to help me sleep better.

From September 2020 to December 2020, I felt moderately okay. My tachycardia improved, but the fainting attacks continued. I was also experiencing a variety of other symptoms—from disturbances in my menstrual cycle (see chapter 9) to debilitating headaches, nausea, chest pain, breathlessness, pins and needles in my toes and fingers, and a buzzing sensation in my head. Tremors soon followed. I continued to look for answers, with the help of my doctor friends and support groups. I was worried but trying to move on, telling myself that I would eventually get better.

Then, in March 2021, nearly a year after my initial infection, I was hospitalized after finding myself unable to stand or stay conscious. Every time I changed positions or tried to walk, I would black out. It was so bad that I could barely stand without support. After a weeklong neurological assessment at the hospital, the doctors determined that I was having an autonomic crisis. I received a diagnosis of Postural Orthostatic Tachycardia Syndrome (POTS)—a term that didn't make a lot of sense to me at the time. Later, I would discover that POTS fell under the dysautonomia umbrella. I was put on steroids and advised to rest in bed at home for three weeks. One of the theories that the neurologist treating me posited was that my POTS and other Long COVID symptoms were being caused by an autoimmune reaction within my body triggered by the initial viral illness. She felt steroid therapy (1 gram of Solu-Medrol for five days followed by a tapered regimen of steroids) could help alleviate my symptoms.

My new diagnosis wasn't surprising, considering my symptoms, but it did leave me very upset. My doctors had told me that there was no cure for dysautonomia, and I went through all five stages of grief over the next few months. Again, I turned to support groups and Dysautonomia International, an organization where I discovered many helpful resources and learned more about what was happening to me.

In April 2021, in the midst of this learning journey, and a few weeks into my steroid treatment—which had provided no relief—I was reinfected with COVID. Since I was on bed rest, my parents had been taking care of me and my child and had moved back in with me. After ten days, my in-laws stepped in to help us out with the care. Little did we know that they had been infected. When they developed their first symptoms, fever and cold, we were alarmed and feared the worst. Unfortunately, my entire family was soon infected, including Rakesh, my parents, and my child. We moved in with my parents to isolate together in their larger house and support one another through this nerve-wracking experience.

For the first six days after testing positive, I barely had any symptoms. Rakesh, my parents, and my child, however, were battling high fevers. Even though I was unable to stand or sit upright for long periods of time, I took on the job of monitoring everyone's vitals.

Outside our home, the situation was quite dire. We were in the midst of India's most devastating COVID wave, which would leave many dead, orphaned, and traumatized. Indians were literally dying from a lack of hospital beds and oxygen. I was receiving news of the deaths of many of my friends' parents and was alarmed. Rakesh's father and uncle were soon admitted to the ICU. People desperate for treatments were trying to buy often unproven medicines on the black market. No one knew what to do.

Then, on the morning of the seventh day after testing positive, I woke up feeling intense pain in my chest and was unable to breathe. I checked my oxygen levels and saw that they were beginning to dip. Just as my family was beginning to recover, I was slipping. I tried lying on my stomach for a few hours—a prone position that had been recommended by doctors for shortness of breath—but my oxygen levels continued to drop. Once they fell below the 90 percent mark, my friend Dr. Sarthak, who had been monitoring our entire family through video calls, said it was time for me to find a hospital bed with oxygen. My father and husband, still quite sick from COVID, began the search and managed to get me admitted to a small hospital nearby.

I was put in the ICU, where I was given oxygen, but the ongoing complications from my POTS seemed to frighten and confuse the doctors treating me. On my third day at that small hospital, my blood pressure shot up so high that it felt like my head was exploding. I was transferred to a bigger hospital where there were neurologists on call, and I stayed in the ICU there for over a week, gasping for breath, fighting for my dear life. I saw many people die in front of me. While I was there, I lost friends to COVID-19, and I know I had many, many praying for me. It is an experience I will never forget, though I sometimes wish I could.

After I was discharged from the hospital, I was grateful for my life but, in many ways, I felt I was back at square one. The POTS symptoms continued, as did every other long-term symptom I'd experienced, and I'd developed new issues from the second infection. On top of my physical symptoms, I was emotionally devastated after having watched so many people die around me in the ICU. It had been exactly one year since my initial infection, but it felt like little progress had been made. It was all too much for me.

There was one thing that was different about my second infection: There was a community waiting for me. A month before I got sick for the second time, I wrote another Twitter thread about my journey of trying to find a diagnosis and the trauma of being denied care by multiple doctors. I described my symptoms in detail and, before I knew it, I was receiving messages from people across the country asking me for advice. While Western countries like the United States and the United Kingdom seemed to have made more progress with regards to Long COVID awareness and research, there was little to no research or conversations about the disease in India. It felt like we were operating in an information vacuum. Patients invariably seemed to know more than doctors and were being forced to advocate for themselves. In many cases, patients were still being dismissed as people with anxiety. After nearly a year seeking medical care and finding most of my answers in support groups, I wasn't entirely surprised.

The support groups I'd been frequenting were crucial to my mental and physical health, but they were based in the UK, the US, and other countries where Long COVID was better recognized. I saw a clear need for community within my own country, which was still in the midst of a deadly wave (and had its own waves of Long COVID), so I decided to create my own group. A few weeks after I was discharged, I started the India Covid Survivors Group on Telegram (now also on Twitter as @longcovidindia) and within days, over two hundred people had joined. At the time of this writing, our group has nearly five hundred members, a small number considering India's population, but we are a vibrant community nonetheless. Every day, we talk about the latest developments in the Long COVID world. Some days, we struggle to cope. But when someone expresses their struggle, we all band together and remind them that they are not alone. We share memes and often use dark humor to cope with the debilitating chronic illnesses many of us are dealing with and the emotions our experiences bring up. We also offer one another logistical support and advice, helping prepare one another for doctor visits and collectively arming ourselves with information on how to self-advocate in medical settings.

I started this group because I realized that the medical establishment, media, and other powerful stakeholders weren't going to solve this problem for us. If doctors were dismissing one of us, that was one too many. Being part of other support groups had helped me immensely in advocating for myself, and I realized how vital peer-to-peer support was. I knew Indian patients needed these resources, too.

Earlier in my career, I spent some years as an advocacy manager for Doctors

Without Borders. This experience taught me that patients often have to advocate for themselves, and as a patient, I knew how difficult this could be—especially in a country as vast as mine or one with competing political interests. Even patient advocates in more "developed" nations were facing the same questions: How do you raise awareness about Long COVID in a country where the government's main focus is individual responsibility, rather than mitigating infection? How do you raise awareness in a country where policymakers are forcing a choice between the economy and public health?

Patient advocacy has always driven change in public health, and I'm not surprised at all that patient support groups and people living with COVID are at the forefront of finding answers about Long COVID. In a global health crisis like the COVID-19 pandemic, we need contributions from a vast range of experts but, most importantly, we need patients' voices. The small community of long-haulers I have built, and am a member of, is following the science more closely than most of the doctors in my country. Many of us have turned this quest for understanding our bodies into a part-time job. In our desire for answers, we have daily conversations about one another's doctors' visits and results and hold one another up when we sense one of us is about to fall. We share research papers, articles, podcasts, and YouTube videos. Many of us have given interviews to national and international media to create awareness about Long COVID in India. We debunk misinformation when we see it and are always on the lookout for like-minded doctors to join our group.

Today, this group includes some health care providers and researchers who patiently answer our queries about the human body and the immune system and advise us on what to do. To me, these health care workers are the medical establishment's best ambassadors. They have been instrumental in helping traumatized patients regain trust in health care providers. Our group also continues to reach out to the medical establishment at large, urging providers to shed their denialism about Long COVID. Some of us have even offered to participate in scientific research and are now in the process of starting our own patient-led research survey, inspired by the work other support groups have done.

As exhausting as all this sounds, it is important for us long-haulers to come together in some form—whether on Facebook, Slack, WhatsApp, another social media platform, or even in-person with members of our local community—and keep speaking up. I am in touch with long-haulers from other parts of South Asia, and the struggle is real, as the research has yet to penetrate our countries. Only patients and peer support groups are driving forward this crucial conversation on Long COVID and related chronic illnesses. We demand our governments do more, policy-wise, and that they allocate funding for research into post-viral illnesses, not just for us, but for everyone in South Asia who has battled a post-viral illness. Talking about Long COVID consistently and continuously not only helps break down stigmas but also helps inform others who may be in need of care or answers. All around the world, patients are gathering, writing, and advocating. Our metaphorical voices reverberate against one another, and grow stronger. Together, we are speaking Long COVID support into existence.

Postscript: As I write this, my POTS symptoms are now manageable and under control thanks to Dr. Sarath Menon, whom I found through Dysautonomia International's website. After months of online consulting, I finally met him in April 2022. He remains among a handful of doctors who are trained in identifying and managing dysautonomia in India. He also confirmed peripheral neuropathy (damage to peripheral nerves), but assured me that I am on a path to healing. What will this healing look like? Only time will tell, but I have hope—for myself and for the millions of us who are now left with bodies that are partially or completely transformed.

Survival Tips

1. **Believe in yourself:** If your gut instinct tells you something doesn't feel right in your body, then you're probably right.

2. **You are not alone:** It may feel like you are, but look for others with similar experiences; use the power of social media to find like-minded communities and groups.

3. **Don't believe everything:** There may be folks in support groups who may claim to have cures, but they're usually trying to cash in on your vulnerability. Google the names of supplements and untested or unregulated herbal remedies (as well as any individuals or companies promoting "cures"). Often, you can easily tell which treatment

suggestions have little-to-no scientific evidence or are being pushed by for-profit companies with murky histories.

4. Understand your body: If you are not a scientist—like I'm not—the quest to understand your body may seem overwhelming, but the internet is filled with fantastic articles, videos, and podcasts that simplify medical terms and explain how our bodies react to infections. I recommend journalist Ed Yong's articles and COVID long-hauler Gez Medinger's YouTube channel. Don't be afraid to utilize these resources or begin a larger journey to understand health and science. Understanding your body will arm you with more information and will help you know (sooner, rather than later) if and when a health care provider is invalidating your claims.

5. Speak up: Share your experiences because it may actually help you find your fellow "spoonies" (see page 266), a term some of us with chronic illnesses call ourselves. You may also help someone else better understand or acknowledge their own long-term symptoms. Speaking up is an excellent way to begin pushing back on the shame and stigma associated with most illnesses, so own your narrative and don't let anyone silence your expression of what you feel.

6. Ask for recommendations: Always ask support groups for health care provider recommendations. In some cases, it may be helpful to ask support group members for reviews of a specific provider you are considering. These conversations may save you from heartbreak and feelings of invalidation. You can also ask support groups for tips on how you can advocate for yourself in various medical settings.

7. Understand your advantages and disadvantages: You may live in a country with more awareness of Long COVID, but a more fractured health care system. You may live somewhere where medical treatments and vaccines have been slow to roll out or are often inaccessible. Stay up-to-date with the news in your area, but also consider connecting with patients in other places to understand how care varies and what you might be able to fight for. Understanding your environment and the tools you have and don't have can be valuable in identifying paths to support and care.

8. Consider all your networks: Patient support groups were a lifeline for me, but so was my network of health journalists and my larger community of family and friends. Without the support of my friend

Dr. Sarthak, I would have lacked answers and support. If you feel comfortable doing so, reach out to family, friends, and professional networks. You never know who might be able to provide help.

9. Make a list of questions for your health care provider and come armed with research: Always go into your appointments prepared to ask questions and demand answers, if need be. Arm yourself with research. You can even send links to your provider in advance if you are already in touch via email or telehealth services. Be humble, but don't let the power imbalance between patient and provider throw you off.

10. Post-ICU PTSD is real: If you've been in the ICU for days or weeks or months, it's possible that you are experiencing post-traumatic stress disorder from your ICU stay. Acknowledge that reality. Accept that you feel the pain and allow yourself to grieve for all that your body, mind, and spirit witnessed, fought for, and survived. It's human to feel as if the ground under you is shaky, and I recommend seeking help from a professional to navigate these feelings. Your trauma is real, but remember that where there is trauma, there can be healing, too.

CHAPTER II

Knowledge Is Power

Navigating Long COVID Research
to Better Understand Your Own Illness

Lisa McCorkell, cofounder of
Patient-Led Research Collaborative

When I got COVID in March 2020, I was in my last semester of graduate school getting my master's in public policy. I was a generalist—someone with an equal interest in all types of policy—and while I took a few classes on health equity (policies that aim to eliminate disparities in health outcomes), I was more interested in social determinants of health than I was in medicine. While my family and I had our fair share of medical issues prior to my developing Long COVID, I was always fairly intimidated by the medical world and was more interested in how policies (and politics) can impact our communities.

One of my main goals in getting my graduate degree was to gain enough quantitative skills to understand whether studies that evaluated different policies were valid. By developing these skills, I would be better equipped to parse research studies—and media articles about research studies—and make sure I never took this information at face value. I wanted to make a positive impact on the world as a government worker, to ensure that my policy decisions were evidence-based, and that the evidence I used was sound and not steeped in bias or ulterior motives.

So, after I was sick with COVID for beyond the two weeks that health agencies and media outlets had promised, I joined the Body Politic COVID-19 support group and offered my new (and slightly underdeveloped) research skills to some members of that group who had developed a survey on lingering and less-well-known symptoms of COVID. Little did I know, that survey and its analysis would be the birth of the Patient-Led Research Collaborative (PLRC), a group of people with Long COVID who have backgrounds in a variety of applicable fields, from machine learning to neuroscience to advocacy, and conduct patient-led research on Long COVID.[1]

As PLRC has conducted our own research, navigated the emerging body of Long COVID research, and immersed ourselves in the body and history of post-viral illness research at large, I've developed the skills necessary to spot when a study is well done and when one is . . . not so well done. Understanding the difference has been truly critical to developing a deeper understanding of my own illness and being able to advocate on behalf of other people with Long COVID and similar illnesses.

Friends of mine have been told by their health care providers not to Google their illnesses, because it will "just cause anxiety." But knowledge is power. When providers try to gatekeep information, they are often taking power away from those most impacted. We deserve to know what is happening to our bodies, to be curious about new findings, and to have agency in the research process and in our own searches for care. This is particularly important for people who have illnesses that are not well understood by the medical community.

You don't need an advanced degree to gain this knowledge, agency, and power. In fact, you are already in possession of some of the most intimate and important knowledge just by having this illness. But being able to learn more about ongoing research can validate your experience—and it can also give you tools you need to advocate for yourself in the doctor's office, with employers, and to your friends and family. Learning about the mechanisms behind Long COVID and potentially helpful treatments can improve your health outcomes. It's important to acknowledge, though, that staying on top of research often requires a certain level of privilege—privileges related to time, energy, stability of symptoms, and cognitive function, and these capacities can vary over time. So, to the extent that you *can* incorporate understanding emerging and ongoing research into your life, I hope this chapter provides you with some of the tools you need to do so successfully.

Navigating Research

The world of research can be daunting. Without an extensive background in academia, it can be difficult to interpret results of a research study from a peer-reviewed article (a scientific paper that has gone through an evaluation process by experts in the field) or a preprint (an earlier version of a scientific paper that is posted online before it goes through a formal peer review process). We often rely on journalists to interpret study results and communicate them to us in an easily digestible way. However, just because a result makes for a catchy headline doesn't mean that the full story is being told. So, let's get into the basics of navigating research so that you can see for yourself if a study on Long COVID is credible.

Types of Studies

When you start looking into biomedical research, you'll come across a few different types of studies. The main ones you'll likely be looking at for Long COVID are as follows.

1. **Studies that characterize an illness:** These studies look at Long COVID symptoms, risk factors, and/or biomedical test results among people with Long COVID, or the pathophysiology of Long COVID, for example.

2. **Studies that evaluate an intervention:** These studies may include therapeutics (for example, a drug's impact on Long COVID symptoms), diagnostics (whether a tool or method can be used to diagnose Long COVID or related illnesses), and prevention (what can help prevent the onset or worsening of Long COVID?).

3. **Studies that measure prevalence:** These studies typically aim to see how common Long COVID is within a specific population, often the general population of a country or humans at large.

4. **Studies that are meta-analyses or systematic reviews:** These studies combine data and findings from multiple studies that all try to answer the same research question.

Locating Studies

But where do you find these studies? Often, research on Long COVID is covered in news articles, shared on social media, or discussed in support groups. However, you can also search directly through online platforms where research is published. Other places to search include the following.

- pubmed.gov: PubMed has over thirty-three million citations for biomedical literature.

- scholar.google.com: Google Scholar includes all types of scholarly literature and academic resources.

- medrxiv.org: This is a preprint server for health sciences. Before an article is peer-reviewed, it will often be posted here so that results can be more quickly disseminated to the public.

In your search, make sure to include other terms for Long COVID used by researchers, like "post-acute sequelae of SARS-CoV-2," "PASC," "post-COVID conditions," and "post-COVID-19 syndrome." Additionally, it may be helpful to search for other diagnoses you've received or that you know are common among people with Long COVID (you can see a list of these on page 141).

Analyzing Studies

Research studies are typically set up with the following structure.

- **Title:** A very brief description of the focus of the paper
- **Authors:** The people who wrote the paper and conducted the research, and their affiliations with universities or organizations
- **Abstract:** Usually a high-level summary of the paper, including the objectives, methods, results, and conclusions. It's typically short, so it often covers very little!
- **Introduction:** Provides context for the research, including research done to date on the topic and what questions the study was aiming to answer.
- **Methods:** Describes how the study was designed and analyzed in detail.
- **Results:** Presents the findings of what was analyzed in the study.
- **Discussion:** Discusses what the findings mean in the context of other studies and patient experience. Also includes the study's strengths and weaknesses, any broader implications, and suggestions for future research.
- **Conclusion:** Wraps the paper up with the big takeaways.
- **Acknowledgments:** Lists the people who helped with the study. Lists sources of funding and any stated conflict of interest.
- **Supplementary Materials:** May include additional text, tables, and graphs that couldn't fit in the main article, like survey questions and more results.

Once you've found a study to review, consider these questions[2]:

- **What is the research question(s)?** (*often found in Introduction*) The research question is what the study is aiming to answer. A good research question will be based on patients' lived experiences and prior research. Look out for research questions that ask something you want to know. Knowing what the research question is will help you decipher the results and determine whether the study answers a useful question.

- **What is the research design?** (*found in Methods*) The research design is how the study was set up. For treatment studies, a randomized control trial (RCT) is considered the gold standard because treatments are randomized, so you can often understand whether a treatment is effective or not based on the treatment itself, and not some confounding variable (like access to health care or types of symptoms). Additionally, if a research study has a control group, the study will be able to compare the group of interest to the control group to see if the group of interest has any significant differences. Again, this doesn't mean that a study that isn't an RCT or doesn't have a control group isn't useful (PLRC's paper was neither, and it helped spark additional research and informed the public on Long COVID), but if it is one or both, results will more likely apply to a larger population. Consider whether the study is quantitative (collects numerical data), qualitative (collects non-numerical data), or a mix of both. A qualitative study could include an analysis of people's experiences, where the researcher identifies common themes across what was shared. Qualitative data provides rich insights where patients can expand on their experiences beyond what a yes-or-no survey or a test result can capture. A study that has a mix of qualitative and quantitative data can be really powerful, with the qualitative data providing crucial context for understanding the quantitative data.

- **Who is in the sample?** (*found in Methods or Results*) The sample is the group of people in the research study. Ideally, a sample should be representative of the broader population of patients with that illness—in terms of demographics, clinical phenotype (how a disease presents itself in an individual), illness trajectory, and illness severity, among others. However, too often samples are not representative. For example, biomedical research is disproportionately conducted on white people[3] and cisgender men,[4] and online surveys exclude people who do not have internet access. Therefore, it's crucial to look at the demographics of the sample studied to see whether the results can be extrapolated to the broader population. If a sample is not representative and does not include all the different types of illness presentations it aims to study, the findings can still be useful, but should be interpreted carefully.

- **How many people are in the sample?** (*found in Methods or Results*) Generally for a quantitative study, the more people in a sample, the more precise the results are. Studies that have a few dozen participants can still be useful, but when there are fewer participants, it becomes less likely that the results of the study can draw conclusions for the rest of the population. For qualitative studies, the sample size is less important, a large sample size is not necessarily needed, as even a few in-depth accounts can provide rich insights and be representative of the target population's experiences (depending on the research question).

- **What is the study measuring?** (*found in Methods and/or Supplementary Materials*) Understanding what the study measured can help determine if the results are comprehensive or just telling part of the story. If the study was survey-based, look at the questions researchers asked to see if they are inclusive and reflective of patients' experiences. A good way to figure this out is to imagine yourself being tasked with answering these questions, and then determine if the questions align well with your experience or not. If the study is reporting lab results, look at the tests they used to see if there may be any missing.

- **What are the findings?** (*found in Results*) Of course, the main point of looking at research studies is to look at the findings! But don't just stick to the abstract section. A finding that may be important and relevant to your experience may be hidden in the results section because it wasn't deemed flashy enough to make the abstract or a big part of the discussion section. Other things to be wary about when reviewing the findings:

  » Researchers choose what findings to share, although best practice is to share all statistically significant results (or even better, all results regardless of significance). Statistical significance measures whether a finding is meaningful, or if it's due to chance.

  » Try to identify whether a result, specifically from treatment studies, is clinically significant as well. Clinical significance aims to understand the size and scope of an effect, so you would be able to better tell if an intervention actually made a meaningful difference for a patient. For example, a study could find that a treatment enabled patients to walk farther than the control group (and the result was statistically significant), but if that distance is a matter of inches, the clinical significance is minimal.

» Relatedly, one of the most important lessons in statistics is that *correlation does not equal causation.* Just because two variables are correlated (for example, variable x increases as variable y increases), does not mean that variable x caused variable y to increase. The authors of the study may have found that two variables correlate and hypothesized that one is causing the other to act in a certain way (often referred to as a "causal relationship"), but unless other variables that could have *also* increased variable y are taken into account, saying variable x caused variable y is inappropriate.

» Though it isn't a frequent occurrence, be aware of "p-hacking," or selective reporting, which is when researchers manipulate results by continuing to conduct statistical tests until they find significance, thereby likely inflating their results. Basically, if you have to run a bunch of different tests in order to prove your hypothesis and only one comes back in your favor, your hypothesis is probably wrong.

- **Who are the authors?** (*found in Authors*) It isn't necessary to be super familiar with the authors of every research study, but it can be helpful to know what their expertise is in, what institution or organization they're associated with, and if they have a reputation within their field. There are unfortunately some bad actors within the research world, who have agendas that aren't in the best interest of patients and may instead be based on professional allegiances or financial interests. Additionally, despite many saying otherwise, every researcher—including me—has internal biases, and those biases may be reflected in research questions, sample size or participant demographics, methods of evaluating results, or the findings that they choose to highlight. Some researchers demonstrate this bias by continuously using research methodology that is not grounded in patient experience and may actually be harmful to the patient community.

- **Who is the study funded by?** (*found in Acknowledgments*) Unfortunately, money can strongly influence research. In some cases, researchers may publish results that are favorable to their funder or can help get a drug into the next phase of a clinical trial. This is not necessarily common, but looking into who is funding a study can help you identify bias based on financial interests or better understand the broader context for the research.

- **Were patients involved in the development of the study?** (*found in Authors, Methods, and/or Acknowledgments*) If patients were involved, it's more likely that the study will be measuring the right things and reflective of patients' experiences. However, even when patients are involved, there are various levels of patient engagement, ranging from tokenizing (including a patient in study development to check a box rather than actively engaging that person's expertise to make the study better) to patient-led (patients are the ones developing, analyzing, and writing the study). Unfortunately, it's often difficult—if not impossible—to decipher the details of patient engagement from a published study. But it is generally a good sign when studies include mention of patient engagement in the methods or acknowledgments section.

So far, I've explained general rules for analyzing and understanding research. But there are a few Long COVID-specific red flags to be wary of when deciphering relevant studies:

- **What is the research question?** Developing a long-term illness after a viral infection is not new. This can happen after contracting many viruses, including the flu, Epstein-Barr virus (EBV), severe acute respiratory syndrome (SARS), and polio. While post-viral illness research has been vastly underfunded over the last several decades, we do have a body of research to start from. Studies on Long COVID should base their research question on existing post-viral illness research, on existing Long COVID research, and on the patient experience.[5] Studies that frame the research question as if the existence of post-viral symptoms is entirely new are not likely to ask the right questions.

- **Who is in the sample?**

  » **If the researchers restrict their definition of people with Long COVID to only those who have had a positive polymerase chain reaction (PCR) COVID test:** PCR tests (the tests that you usually get at a health care provider or testing center) are considered the "gold standard" for detecting COVID. But these tests have sometimes been difficult for patients to access, notably during the first waves of the pandemic, when tests were not yet widely available, and during surges, when demand can overwhelm supply. According to a study in *Nature*, during the first wave, only 1 to 4 percent of all COVID cases were confirmed.[6] As of September 2021, the Centers for Disease Control and Prevention in the United States estimated that only 25 percent of all COVID cases had been reported.[7] Additionally, PCR tests are most accurate when administered at the exact right time after exposure—not too early, not too late. In PLRC's published study—which analyzed survey results from people who became sick prior to June 2020, only 15.9 percent of respondents had received a positive PCR or antigen ("rapid") test result. The remaining people either had not been able to access a test or had tested negative, likely because they weren't tested at the right time. In fact, the primary difference we found between people who tested positive and those who tested negative was *when* they were tested (day six of illness for those who tested positive, day forty-three for those who tested negative). When comparing symptom prevalence between the two groups, we found no statistically significant difference in all but 2 out of 203 symptoms.[8] Therefore, Long COVID studies that include anyone who reports Long COVID symptoms, regardless of having a positive PCR test, will have more representative findings.

» **If researchers restrict their definition of people with Long COVID to only those who have COVID antibodies:** One way researchers have tried to address PCR testing accessibility and accuracy issues is by relying on COVID antibodies to determine whether someone has Long COVID or not. The studies that use this method include people who do not have COVID antibodies in a control group (which is supposed to be a group of people who do not have the illness and are studied in comparison to those who do). Unfortunately, this methodology is flawed. Several studies have demonstrated that having lower levels of antibodies can actually be an indicator that someone has Long COVID.[9] Demographics matter here as well: Patients who have higher levels of antibodies tend to be male, of an older age, and/or people who were hospitalized in the acute phase of their COVID infection.[10] When reviewing research, be wary of any study that claims to be studying Long COVID but uses the presence of COVID antibodies to determine whether or not someone has Long COVID.

» **If they're only studying hospitalized patients:** Often, researchers studying COVID outcomes only look at hospitalized patients. However, several studies have shown that many people with Long COVID were never hospitalized during their acute illness.[11] In our study, for example, that number was 91.6 percent.[12] While it is critical for hospitalized patients to be studied as well, study samples should reflect that distribution when trying to characterize and treat Long COVID.

• **What is the study measuring?** In Long COVID research, post-exertional malaise (the worsening of existing or appearance of new symptoms 12 to 48 hours following any kind of exertion) is too often not asked about as a symptom, despite it being one of the top three symptoms our survey respondents reported.[13] Many studies that attempt to track the prevalence of Long COVID ask respondents about a very limited set of symptoms, often leaving out important ones like neurological/cognitive symptoms and instead focusing on respiratory symptoms. Studies with short or narrow symptom lists are bound to not capture everyone with Long COVID. As a reminder, PLRC tracked 203 symptoms, and that likely doesn't even capture all the symptoms associated with Long COVID.

This is a lot of information to keep track of, and I didn't even mention everything! If you're still not confident in your ability to decipher a complex research study, or if you're questioning the results or methodology of a study you've seen featured in the news, it can be helpful to turn to Twitter, Reddit, or a Long COVID support group to see if others have summarized the results of or issues with the study. Copying the link to the article and pasting it in the search bar on Twitter can help you find these threads, or you can go directly to trusted sources to see if they've covered it.[14] However, it's still important to understand who is writing the summary and what their biases may be.

Understanding Your Own Illness

Understanding the trends and new insights emerging from ongoing research can be very helpful for learning more about your own illness, but everyone experiences illness differently. With Long COVID, which likely has several different causes and mechanisms, it's important to understand the trajectory of your own illness. Collecting data on yourself can help you identify triggers, be able to rest and pace better, and help your health care providers understand what your illness looks like over time instead of only on the day that they see you. Different ways to learn more about your illness include the following:

1. Tracking your symptoms, triggers, and treatments. With an illness like Long COVID, where post-exertional malaise, fatigue, and cognitive dysfunction are the three most common symptoms, you may find that the cognitive effort it takes to track symptoms is simply too much to do regularly. I suggest making this process as easy as possible, by documenting symptoms in whatever way works for you, and asking a caregiver/loved one to help you. Examples of how you can track your illness include the following:

    -   Google Form: You can create a Google Form that lists symptoms, triggers, diet, activities, treatments, and more, and at the end of each day, you or a caregiver or loved one can fill out the form, indicating the symptoms you experienced that day, what activities you did, what treatments you tried, and what triggers you experienced.

    -   App: There are many apps that can help you track your symptoms. Make sure to choose one that is customizable so that you can add your own symptoms or other unique aspects to your illness.

    -   Journal: If you're not technologically savvy, don't have regular access to the internet or a smartphone, or have difficulties tolerating screen time, journaling about your symptoms and triggers can work just as well!

2. If you can afford one, consider using a wearable device like a Garmin or Fitbit.

    -   Wearable devices can track your heart rate and heart rate variability, which can be crucial for managing POTS and other autonomic symptoms. Garmin also has a Body Battery feature that can help you identify when you need to rest throughout the day based on your activity and stress levels, helping you pace and prevent post-exertional malaise.

Identifying trends in symptom severity, triggers, and what treatments help or make symptoms worse is a way of doing your own research! Your body is providing the data you can use to make informed decisions about activity management and what the right treatments for you may be. By collecting this data on yourself, you can also report trends to your community and assist in research efforts on Long COVID.

Getting Involved in Research

PARTICIPANT

A great way to help in making discoveries is to be part of a research study yourself. To find a research study to participate in:

- Ask your health care providers if they are aware of any studies you can be part of.

- Keep an eye out for recruitment posts in support groups and on social media.

- Sign up for mailing lists that publicize research studies—PLRC and Solve ME both do so, and their newsletters can be accessed at patientresearchcovid19.com and solvecfs.org/news-and-insights/subscribe-to-newsletter.

- If you're in the United States, you can search for trials that are recruiting at clinicaltrials.gov.

When determining which studies you should sign up for, you'll want to consider many of the same questions I suggested for reviewing research. Knowing what the research question is, who the authors are, who the study is funded by, who is included in the sample, what the research design is, and whether patients have been involved in the development of the study can help you determine if the study is going to be worth your time and energy.

And there are additional important considerations:

- **If the study involves any type of medical testing, will you receive the results?** Receiving results of testing, like blood tests and imaging, is one of the biggest incentives to participating in research because many tests can otherwise be difficult to access. Co-pays for tests can be high, and private insurance doesn't always cover them. For people who are uninsured, tests can be outrageously unaffordable. Additionally, it can be difficult to get health care providers to order you some of the less commonly understood tests. In these situations, getting these tests done for free by participating in a research study can be hugely beneficial for you and can help you understand your illness better, at no financial cost. However, some studies may not share your test results with you, and the other costs of being part of the study (like the exertion it may take) may be too high to not have ownership over data you provide to a study. Consider all of these factors when deciding if you'd like to participate.

- **What are the risks to you?** Understand that there may be risks to participating in the study. For example, there may be side effects of a new treatment, or a test that requires exertion may cause a severe crash, so it is important to talk to your health care provider about the potential benefits and risks of participation. Additionally, ask about the study's data sharing practices to ensure your data is secure and not being shared with third parties without your consent.

- **What is required of you to participate?** Look into what the time and energy commitment is like, and think seriously about whether participation for you would be feasible: Will participating involve a lot of trips to the lab or to a research institution that is several hours away? Do you have the ability to get there? If not, can the research team provide transportation? Will you be compensated for your time? If the study is a survey, how long do the researchers estimate it will take respondents to complete it, and are you able to stop to rest and come back to it later?

Making a decision to be part of a research study always requires weighing the costs against the benefits. There can be immense benefits—for yourself, for your community, for society—but sometimes the cost—to your health, finances, or schedule—may be too high. It can be helpful to talk through these decisions with your loved ones, your community, and a trusted health care provider if you have one.

PATIENT REPRESENTATIVE

A step beyond being a participant in a study is to be a patient representative, representing the patient experience to the researchers conducting the study and helping to shape the study. Being a patient representative can be a great way to contribute to science and to your community because you can help ensure the study is focusing on what patients need and want answers to. With roots in the HIV/AIDS crisis in the late 1980s, the practice of engaging those with lived experience in the development of study design and analysis has become more and more prevalent.

To get involved, keep your eyes open for calls for patient representatives. If you are already enrolled in a study, ask what the researchers' engagement with patients looks like and whether patients can contribute to the study design. Keep in mind that helping to inform the design and analysis of a research study should always be a paid position; you are providing both your lived experience with the illness and all of your skills to better the study, and you should be compensated accordingly. The National Health Council has a Fair Market Value Calculator you can use to determine how much you should be getting paid for your contributions.[15]

If you're chosen as a patient representative, connect with other patient representatives on the study so you can support one another and raise any concerns together. Ask the study coordinators for what you need to be successful in this role, and be sure to advocate for yourself and for your community in all decision-making spaces.

RESEARCHER

Often, traditional medical research does not provide people with answers quickly enough. While our lives, livelihoods, and quality of life hang in the balance, nimbleness and expediency are not hallmarks of academia. There are reasons for this: Researchers want to make sure research is conducted ethically, is representative, and is methodologically sound. However, when patients are in crisis, we need answers fast, and sometimes the best way to get these answers is to do research on your community yourself.

Conducting patient-led research can take a variety of forms.

- Informal polls: If you have a hypothesis you're interested in and you're part of a support group, you can post an informal poll to test that hypothesis (while understanding the limitations of who you are polling—in sample size and demographics).[16]

- Traditional research: If you are able to receive Institutional Review Board (IRB) or ethics approval, you can conduct a study that can be accepted in a peer-reviewed journal, which can give the research more legitimacy in the eyes of academics. During the COVID pandemic, preprints have become more commonly accepted and covered by news outlets. Preprints are useful because we get to see researchers' findings earlier, but we also have to be more rigorous in deciphering studies that are not yet peer-reviewed. For example, PLRC's second survey had ethics approval from University College London; our results were first posted as a preprint on medRxiv in December 2020 and were then peer-reviewed and published in the *Lancet's eClinicalMedicine*.[17] Even when our work was still a preprint, it provided people with important information about Long COVID while we waited for the peer-review process to finish. People with Long COVID were able to better understand their own health and help their doctors do so, too; researchers were able to form research questions based on our findings and start on their own research.

- Other: Patients have found ways to conduct their own research in many other ways; for example, people with diabetes have constructed a new mobile technology system and people with amyotrophic lateral sclerosis (ALS) have conducted their own treatment trial.[18]

It's also important to understand the limitations of extrapolating results. A lot of patient-led research is limited in scope due to lack of funding, and the results cannot necessarily be extrapolated to the entire patient population. However, when we need answers now, even small polls can be very helpful for getting a pulse on what is happening, and they can lead to additional hypotheses and guide future research.

Overall, while it can be difficult to decipher whether a study is credible and is applicable to you, research is a tool you can use to learn more about your illness and to educate others (including your health care provider). Over time, you may get better at understanding and using research. To the extent that you or a caregiver are able to, being aware of new research, tracking symptoms, and being involved in research can be empowering. It can help us all come to a better collective understanding of Long COVID.

Survival Tips

Navigating Long COVID research can be daunting, but when you know how to best approach it, it can become a powerful tool that can assist you in your health journey. When reviewing a research study, if you're able to answer the following questions, you'll have a good understanding of what the study found, if it is credible, and if the results are applicable to you:

What is the research question?

What is the research design?

Who is in the sample?

How many people are in the sample?

What is the study measuring?

What are the findings?

Who are the authors?

Who is the study funded by?

Were patients involved in the development of the study?

Beyond reviewing research, joining a research study as a participant or patient representative, as well as being a researcher yourself, can help you better understand Long COVID and provide you and your community with needed answers.

CHAPTER 12

Such a Powerful Love

Disabled and Chronically Ill People and Our Long Fight for Justice

JD Davids and Naina Khanna

Being sick, especially chronically ill, can be an incredibly isolating experience—perhaps that's why it can feel so tremendously healing when we come together in community with others who have shared experiences. Disabled and chronically ill people have long taken action to care for ourselves and one another, to demand that our lived experiences are recognized and that systems that affect us respond to them. There are so many ways this can happen, all valuable—from sharing tips on coping emotionally and managing symptoms, to collaborating on acts of resistance against biased health care providers or ableist structures, to participating in mutual aid efforts to care for one another and global campaigns to demand access to lifesaving treatments.

This book is an important addition to a long legacy of chronically ill people sharing information, finding our own answers and organizing for justice in our own lives and in the world around us. As two chronically-ill people—one living with HIV, the other with Long COVID and other complex chronic conditions—we welcome you to this community and thank you for all you have already done to take care of yourself. We also take this opportunity to share our stories with you—in the hope that these anecdotes of advocating for ourselves and others may provide you with useful historical context, a sense of camaraderie, and guidance for what may lay ahead.

Long COVID advocacy started just weeks into the pandemic, as many with COVID realized they weren't getting better and were facing disbelief from others at every turn. Long COVID, and the advocacy it spurred, is unique in the sense that it developed during a particular time in global history and in the history of economics of research and medicine, and in a specific political context. But Long COVID advocacy is also part of a long and powerful trajectory of chronically ill and disabled people realizing they had to advocate for themselves, and in doing so, finding a community to advocate with. This work has changed so many things for the better—from public policies and programs around illness and disability to the conduct and funding of research and medical care, and, crucially, the individual lives of countless disabled and chronically ill people like us.

We—the coauthors of this chapter—are comrades who met early in the millennium as fellow travelers in social justice movements in the United States. Naina (she/they) is a forty-five-year-old South Asian, caste-privileged, cisgender, daughter of immigrants, living with HIV since 2002. JD (he/him) is a fifty-four-year-old disabled, white, queer, and trans person of Ashkenazi Jewish descent, living with ME/CFS and several other complex chronic conditions, now including Long COVID.

We deepened our relationship as two collaborators in the 2008 founding of Positive Women's Network USA (PWN), a national network of women and people of trans experience living with HIV, where Naina currently serves as codirector. PWN fights for human rights and dignity for people living with HIV, using a racial, gender, and economic justice lens. JD is a long time HIV and health justice activist who is now bringing these experiences into current efforts as one of the founders of the Network for Long COVID Justice.

We see many parallels in the struggles of people living with HIV and people living with Long COVID—and also parallels in themes and strategies of resistance. Many people living with HIV, like those living with Long COVID, have faced stigma and discrimination, judgment and bias, and they deal with symptoms that may not always be visible but which may require accommodations. In this chapter, we hope to share some of our personal experiences and learnings from HIV and health justice advocacy that may be relevant to people living with Long COVID.

Before we dive in, we want to provide a bit more information on our perspectives. We each come to this work with a different set of life experiences and learnings. We carry significant privileges; both of us may be understood by others as nondisabled or not seen as chronically ill, as neither of us currently uses mobility or communication aids, and we both benefit from having income and family resources that allow us to avoid the significant challenges of public assistance or needing home services and support. We also wish to acknowledge what the power of generationally passed down wisdom has done for us and the brilliance of beloved movement ancestors, including Marco Castro-Bojorquez and PWN-USA cofounder Loren Jones, who both died in 2021.

For both of us, the HIV group WORLD (Women Organizing to Respond to Life-Threatening Diseases) was a big influence. It was founded in the 1990s as a peer support and advocacy organization by and for women living with HIV in an era when women-specific AIDS conditions were not even legitimated. We've never forgotten WORLD's slogan: *You are not alone.* We want everyone finding their way with Long COVID to know that you, too, are not alone, and you are loved.

For many of us, our relationships with other disabled and chronically ill people are essential to our well-being, as they are rooted in a powerful and specific love. People with Long COVID are fighting for rapid creation of large-scale programs of services, treatment, and care, but we also need access to support from one another. There's never *not* a need for what people with Long COVID call *patient-led efforts*. Following decades of advocacy, the HIV community has a relatively robust set of programs and treatment for HIV, but we still *deeply* need spaces centered on relationships, community building, and support in the HIV community.

As disabled and chronically ill people, we understand in ways that others may not. We do not give up on one another, and we do not forget that so many of the challenges we face come not from our own conditions but from a disabling society that doesn't prioritize our ease, access, rest, or peace. Community care is essential for our wellness; indeed, it is core to visioning our liberation.

Although we're not always able to be physically together for every conversation (we, the coauthors, live on different coasts and haven't seen each other in-person since the pandemic began), our dialogue continues. We like to think that despite our geographic distance, we are always in-person in a sense—we bring all of ourselves through the screen, the phone, or onto the page, with the full force of our love. To transparently share what this sort of deeply rich and supportive relationship can look like, we've decided to tell our story in the form of a transcript, based on a conversation we started on Zoom video and continued through email in January and February 2022. We've edited it for clarity, accuracy, and length.

JD: All right, so here we are on Dr. King's birthday, which seems somewhat apropos. I thought we could start off by talking about—concisely, but vividly—our memories of first coming to awareness about our chronic conditions, and then into advocacy spaces led by people living with HIV.

I've been chronically ill my whole life, really, though my family and I never named it as such—in part because nothing was severe or life-threatening. Whatever may be the root cause, I have a strange immune system that is too active in some ways and not vigilant enough in others. When I look back now, I can see how my frequent bouts of viral and bacterial infections and relentless allergies changed so many things about my life and relationships, like frequently missing school. I can now see how being a sickly kid heightened the feelings of difference and fear of judgment I carried as someone who was already one of the few Jews in the community and who was puzzled by gender expectations I didn't really identify with.

I came into the HIV activist group ACT UP when I was finishing college in 1990. I was starting to have glimmers of queerness in myself, realizing what I had long suppressed. And I was trying to find a way to do good in the world around me. Then my friend Mike brought me to an ACT UP meeting, and I was put to work.

There wasn't a question about whether to center the people who were most affected, because people living with HIV had started the group. It was an activist group that did things, but it really at the heart was a community and a home, so that's always, always stayed with me. For the first time in my life, I was around people for whom illness was the norm, not the exception. And, in a way, difference itself was the norm—we were a crew of sick people and allies, queer people, current and former drug users, and others who were drawn together by a virus and a commitment to doing all we could to save ourselves, our loved ones, our friends.

Naina: That's so beautiful. I was diagnosed with HIV in 2002, and it came as a shock. I dealt with a lot of internalized stigma and shame and really didn't know how to talk about it or manage this diagnosis for a while. I also didn't have health care—this was before the Affordable Care Act—and insurance companies could legally discriminate against you based on preexisting conditions. So, I was kind of terrified to even get initial bloodwork done to find out how I was doing—viral load, CD4 count, et cetera. I didn't get bloodwork done until

236 · The **LONG COVID** Survival Guide

nearly two years after my initial diagnosis and, during that time, I had a great community of friends and a wonderful family, but I really didn't have any support specifically around dealing with my HIV status. The first time I did go to get bloodwork done, it wasn't a great experience. My numbers weren't as good as I expected them to be, and the doctor wanted me to start meds right away. I wasn't ready, and I also had a lot of questions about the potential implications of treatment regimens if I were to get pregnant. The (white, cis, male) providers dismissed or didn't answer these concerns. So, I left that experience and really didn't pursue HIV care or treatment for another year.

In 2005, I moved to California and found WORLD. Then I was in a community of women, primarily women of color, living with HIV who had self-organized to create the kinds of systems and services they needed.

That experience was transformative for me. I was a person living with HIV who was resisting getting on medication. And I had a peer advocate who was completely nonjudgmental, totally understood my experience, and had some understanding of my spirituality. She understood my concerns about disclosure and confidentiality, and that I was living in a house with a bunch of roommates who didn't know about my HIV status. I had so many walls up around my own disclosure, and accessing care and treatment. And she would just check on me regularly, call me, no pressure. I kept coming up with excuses for why I couldn't go into the office to meet with her. And she would say, "Okay, well, I just got this new issue of this treatment magazine, and it has all the latest medications on it. And I thought you might be interested. Can I get it to you?" And I was like "No, no, no. . . ." And then she finally said, "I'm gonna drop it off at your house in an unmarked envelope." And that worked.

So, I got connected to this community of WORLD, which had been created in a kitchen by and for women living with HIV. We were designing, implementing, and executing programs in ways that really worked for folks. And so that's how I really started to understand the power of spaces that are set up to respond to cultural, gender, racial, and ethnic nuances of our lives, services that are designed by and for folks who are most directly impacted. It was not only transformative for my own experience, it was also the gateway to me getting more involved in HIV organizing and activism, because everyone deserves this. Health care and related systems are usually set up with the particular lens of those who hold power, which historically in the US has mostly been cis, white men with class privilege. We all have a right to spaces and services that are created by us and for us. This stance is what led to the founding of HIV organizations like WORLD and Christie's Place for women, Thrive SS for Black gay men in the South, and so many other groups, many of which have sadly disappeared off the landscape today due to funding challenges—with devastating consequences for the communities they served.

JD: I can imagine that woman, and all she did, because I've known so many people living with HIV, who—in the most firm and gentle way at the same time—are so patient and persistent in their peer support. I wish that could reach everyone with Long COVID and other complex chronic conditions—that depth of connection and caring and acceptance.

I've seen such incredible acceptance—not always without flaws and limits and people having their own biases and things, of course. But I've seen such intense connections between people who came from very different walks of life, and very different backgrounds, bridging the experiences. I've seen—let's say—a straight, cisgender grandma, and a young, gender-expansive queer kid, both living with HIV, who met over that commonality and came together to understand each other and fight with and for each other. They may not have encountered each other otherwise, especially if they are of different races, in this heavily segregated country.

Naina: Yes, totally. I've seen those common experiences just breaking down all kinds of barriers. And really opening minds, opening hearts.

JD: The mentorship was incredible. I have a clear memory of Kiyoshi Kuromiya, who came to the HIV movement after a long history in the civil rights and gay liberation movements, teaching us about how when someone's in the hospital and they need clean sheets, you just go and you find the sheets, and you bring them to the room. You can get assistance (if the hospital staff has time), but you always relate with compassion and practicality to both the hospital staff and the patient in the room. They're all on the team, and they all are to be treated as if they're in it together, with common cause.

And we'd just do what we needed to do. Kiyoshi would be sitting next to Dr. Fauci one day, and the next, he'd be in the hospital, making sure someone had ice chips, or whatever it was. You just did what needed to be done.

When we come together as people facing a disease or health challenge, across our different communities and life experiences, we can share information and approaches that can help us all. For example, in the history of the HIV pandemic, people who came together in the activist group ACT UP included a whole bunch of lesbians who'd been part of the women's health movement, which was about a very embodied understanding of their own bodies. They had the experience of literally taking matters into their own hands, using speculums and flashlights to learn what their cervixes looked like, while at the same time critiquing how medical establishments talked about gender, women, reproduction, and sex.

And so, this sort of do-it-yourself, DIY practice—from which we can learn about our bodies and health even as we work to change bias and stigma in the health care system—came to ACT UP, allowing people of all genders to feel more confident in speaking up about what our bodies needed.

Today, people are sharing a range of experiences within patient-led Long COVID groups to help care for ourselves and one another. I see what people are bringing to it, even with the pandemic constraints that we may have. I recognize it from that intense HIV connection, and now I see it with people living with Long COVID.

As I said, I've been chronically ill for a long time, and for the last fifteen years, that's included experiencing some scarier symptoms, lasting disability, and a range of diagnoses that now many people with Long COVID are getting. And having had COVID twice now, some of my conditions became worse thanks to Long COVID.

When I came to the Body Politic support group, I actually learned from people with Long COVID about mast cell activation syndrome, and a new range of treatments I could try. This was *never* discussed with me by the myriad specialists I've seen over the years, and it's been rapidly and deeply helpful in reducing my pain, helping my digestion, and zapping my brain fog—so much that I was able to resume full-time work for the first time in years! In return, I've shared about less-common treatments for fatigue that I've found helpful as a person with ME/CFS. That's the kind of magic that happens in patient-led movements.

Naina: I don't think we can talk about these dynamics of peer support and the lineage of activism in the HIV movement without talking about the Denver

Principles in 1983, which was kind of the "Bill of Rights" for people living with HIV. This was a seminal moment in HIV organizing—gay men living with AIDS got up on a stage at the fifth annual Gay and Lesbian Health Conference in Denver and read a manifesto demanding the right to a voice in decision-making on the HIV research, care, and treatment agenda, to be treated with full respect and dignity, and to be recognized as experts in their own right. The Denver Principles are an important part of the embodied health social movement's lineage. In claiming legitimacy from an embodied perspective, people with HIV were building off a legacy of Black Panther Party clinics, feminist health praxis, and the idea that those who are directly impacted can take care of one another when nobody else would.

Isolation is a common experience across HIV and COVID. What do you do when you get or might have COVID? You're told to isolate, right? The pandemic has been such an isolating experience for so many people, for obvious reasons, which reminds me of the early days of HIV in some ways. There was so much fear, misinformation, stigma, and just such a lack of awareness about transmission. People with HIV/AIDS were literally cast out by their families and communities or suffered in silence alone because they were afraid to tell anyone. And that hasn't really gone away! There are still folks being forced to eat off of paper plates because those around them think that HIV could be transmitted through surfaces, or who don't get to see certain family members, even today.

People living with HIV looked out for one another when nobody else would. I see a lot of parallels with that in the Long COVID movement and with COVID survivors organizing. I've seen and observed folks documenting their symptoms from the early days, starting to build a repository and conduct their own community-based research on what was happening even when they were being gaslit and told Long COVID was not a thing.

People living with HIV did the same thing. HIV activists were saying that there will be nothing about us, without us. There will be no research trials without our involvement in thinking through what those trials look like. This continues to be important, and we still have to push for it in HIV research, all these years later. For example, people with HIV who menstruate have been gaslighted and told there is no research basis around menopause symptoms appearing to come earlier and maybe more severely. This is, in part, because the people who are making decisions about what to research and which research is valuable in the context of living with HIV are largely people who do not menstruate and do not live with HIV.

These are radical interventions to make in a space where scientific knowledge is still emerging, in a relentlessly capitalist society where health is so tied to ideas of productivity, and where we're told that there are certain types of medical knowledge and research knowledge that are important and others that are not.

That's why we also need to be engaged as decision makers on decisions that are going to impact our lives. This is especially true for people in communities that are historically marginalized from decision-making, from setting priorities for an agenda, or from leadership—usually due to race, ethnicity, gender, gender identity, poverty, lack of formal education, and other structural barriers. Today, all these years later, people with HIV are still fighting to have lived experience at the center of policies, programs, and care. In the HIV context, we are demanding that quality of life for people living with HIV really matters, in its own right. That success for us cannot simply be measured by the quantity of HIV in our bloodstreams; it's also about our emotional and mental health. Do we have enough food to eat? Are we housed? Can we financially survive? Do we have social support? These are also considerations for many people dealing with Long COVID as outlined in other chapters in this book.

JD: "Quality of life" is such a deep thing, and it can be so distant and overlooked in medical care. At the core, it's about what is most meaningful to each person. When we have complex chronic illnesses, we often don't get much support in formal medical settings to think through and identify for ourselves what's most important. For years, I experienced a queasy dizziness that none of my providers wanted to prioritize, but I came to realize it was one of the most persistent factors in my life affecting my ability to work, to parent and to tend to my emotional wellness. Eventually, I started repeatedly demanding referrals to those who might be able to help, and I was referred to a Vestibular Rehabilitation Center; within weeks, the dizziness was mostly gone and my life felt so much more like my own again. But, if I had never spoken up or pushed back against the answers I was repeatedly being given, I never would have experienced that improvement in my quality of life.

My ability to be vocal and persistent about my priorities like this is because of the loving mentorship of my role models in health justice—particularly women living with HIV, trans people, and people with complex chronic conditions like ME/CFS. It's like I have an invisible cheerleading squad inside me that keeps me pushing for what I need, so I don't feel alone.

Disability Justice

JD: I want to talk about disability justice, because I hope it will be baked into the DNA of Long COVID advocacy in ways that that didn't happen with HIV, where there was a distancing, even an othering, around disability.

For years, I'd heard people living with HIV say, "but we're not disabled," as a call for recognition of their worth and humanity. Then in the 2020 film *Crip Camp*, which was otherwise so inspiring, one of the disability rights protest leaders says, "But we're not sick!" on the mic, seeking to do the same thing. So, these roots are long and gnarly.

Those disability rights activists fought for and won legal protections and recognition of disabled people. But we know that having theoretical legal or civil rights doesn't dismantle the injustices of white supremacy, gender bias, and anti-immigrant practices that affect so many disabled people. So now, *disability justice*, which was first named by a collective of queer disabled people of color called Sins Invalid, is moving us beyond rights to liberation—with practices and principles that are deeply intersectional, rooted in and dedicated to the worthiness of all. But still, it doesn't mean that the HIV community has necessarily followed that same trajectory. Even though it's a health justice movement, I feel that there's a lot of stigma about disability in the HIV community, where there's often bias against people who are less healthy and less able-bodied—and often not enough discussion about accessibility, for example. What's your take on that?

Naina: The long-term survivors movement in HIV, and many of the organizing spaces that are created by people living with HIV, rely on various principles of disability justice, but I don't think it's always explicitly named. On the other hand, there's a reason we refer to something called "AIDS, Inc."—the idea that entire careers, institutions, and pharmaceutical companies have been built on the suffering of people living with HIV. People have built careers and institutions on the HIV epidemic, while making invisible critical contributions from, needs of, and leadership from Black people, transgender women, and communities of color—without whom we literally wouldn't be here today.

Race, class, and capitalism, including internalized capitalism—the idea that a person's worth relates to their productivity—white supremacy, and an increasing takeover of advocacy and organizing funding by large pharmaceutical companies, continue to shape how people with chronic conditions are perceived and treated. Ableism is very connected to a capitalist view of the world. We are all living inside of capitalism.

And I think that that very much relates to other kinds of power and privilege in terms of the people who were seen as the faces of the HIV movement in the early days, who were portrayed and visible—it was primarily cisgender, white men in affluent cities, like New York and San Francisco, where there was a lot of access to media resources, positional power, and proximity to political power. I see the disability justice movement as being—from the start—much more intersectional and much more visibly driven by BIPOC folks.

JD: Yeah, and what happened in HIV under capitalism is that it's not just a virus or a disease, it's a *market*, a huge market—and honestly, Long COVID will be, too. The messaging from the market and from the government is that people with HIV should focus on wellness and health, which are great things to have access to when you've been told you likely have a death sentence. But when the first effective combination treatment for HIV emerged, the photos in the ads were often of mountain hikers or athletic bikers, even though that wasn't feasible for many people, even when they got on a lifesaving treatment.

People are encouraged to think of themselves as successfully living with conditions or health challenges in *opposition to disability,* not as disabled people successfully finding their way in a biased and inaccessible society that fears and shames sickness. And this is extra thorny when we realize that many people with Long COVID may have been chronically ill or disabled pre-pandemic. For those of us for whom this is true, will our experiences be seen as less important than those newly disabled or sick from Long COVID?

To do "well" is to repudiate disability, and actual illness is taken as a sign of weakness, failure, or personal decision making gone awry. So, it makes it even more challenging to find that common cause, even though the most inevitable thing that will happen to all of us, if we're lucky, is that we will age, and we will become chronically ill, and we will be living with disabilities or disabled. *But that is seen as the problem*, in this ableist society.

So, you have the early days of the HIV movement concurrent with the super powerful direct action movement of disabled people that won the Americans with Disability Act (ADA) that people with HIV have been very much benefited from. I feel our communities have been pushed apart from each other. Yes, because of funding, and also because it's the marketing of ableism that we're all individuals striving for "wellness," and thus even our health movements can be incredibly ableist.

In #MEAction, an organization I serve on the board of, we advocate as and for people with ME/CFS. And our members have extremely limited energy and capacity and are super marginalized—that's why we're constantly looking for ways for people to give input online or share their stories through art or song if that's accessible for them. We bring photos of our most severely ill folks to our annual Millions Missing mobilization, since they can't physically attend. We have community events where people can watch a film together online, from our beds, if we're up for it. There's an annual Severe ME Day where we especially center and draw attention to those who are the most severely affected; but every single day, we need to understand how to overcome ableism in our own efforts so we're not marginalizing our own people.

Naina: I think that's right on about the HIV movement. For as long as I've been part of it, it hasn't really had a critique of capitalism. There are so many internalized narratives among people living with HIV, as you're pointing to, about productivity and well-being.

For example, something that I've heard a lot, and continue to hear, is people really making big distinctions between HIV and AIDS. People living with HIV often are really proud to say, "Oh, I've been living with HIV, but I don't have AIDS. I've never had AIDS. I'm not one of those people." That distancing: "I'm not one of *those* people." In reshaping self-identity after a life-transforming diagnosis, it can become really important to try to preserve *something*, whatever it is, even when it comes at the cost of oppressing others, in ways that may not always be obvious.

This is also super complicated, because access to resources that allow us to survive in both the US and globally have often been tied to markers of sickness, like services that you can only access if your immune system's T cells are below a certain number. Globally, there have been guidelines for antiretroviral therapy that require T Cells below 200 or 350 to qualify for lifesaving medications that are being produced for a fraction of the cost of what they are sold for. When mine were below 200, a housing case manager advised me to get paperwork in real quick before starting meds. I wonder if there may be markers and limits like this for Long COVID? I know there have already been challenges, with some people not being able to get into some Long COVID clinics because they don't have a documented positive COVID test.

It's very complex—the intersections of individualism and independence and capitalism and human dignity, the ways that capitalism literally requires people to be sick and poor in order to survive, and how we cognitively seek to thrive and gain a sense of self while living with a chronic illness that is so deeply stigmatized, even criminalized.

JD: With Long COVID, this ableist framework will show up as stigma for those who don't "recover," as if it's a mark of personal failing. We're going to see how false differences, or small differences, or misinterpreted, exaggerated differences will play into judgment about who is doing the right thing to fix their Long COVID and being productive and working at it, and who's not.

Who's to blame, who are we talking about when we say someone "fails" a treatment? That's not it—the treatment failed you. And often, the whole system fails you, when it comes to rampant anti-Blackness and other forms of bias in health care. Complex chronic conditions are so underfunded and marginalized in medicine that even white people with private insurance often can't get a diagnosis or good care a lot of the time. But it's much harder for Black and brown people to even find out they have a complex chronic condition, which is also fed by and furthers destructive myths like ME/CFS supposedly being a privileged white woman's disease. I've seen similar misguided assumptions made about Long COVID.

We're neither failures for being sick nor guilty or to blame for getting a health condition. That's the importance of the HIV activist slogan "All people with AIDS are innocent."[1] There was a whole "innocent victim" message about babies born with HIV, for example, and we needed to say that all people living with HIV are innocent, in terms of deserving health care and rights.

I hope people with Long COVID reading this conversation know that this sort of blame is entirely misplaced, and that if they witness it or experience it, they can speak or write about why this is problematic and can harm all of us—once you start drawing lines between "deserving" and "undeserving," we all are at risk of exclusion and harm.

We're already seeing judgment about how people get COVID, even though it's an incredibly easy-to-get airborne virus. I feel strongly that it's also dangerous and counterproductive to shun unvaccinated people who get COVID or Long COVID. One main reason people took longer to get vaccinated or haven't gotten the vaccine is that they don't have a trusted provider. And others have very real histories of first developing ME/CFS symptoms or of these conditions worsening after vaccination, so it's not such an easy decision for those among us who have had those experiences. I know some folks in the Long COVID community have similarly experienced setbacks after vaccination and feel the topic is too stigmatized to discuss publicly. Lumping chronically ill folks in with anti-vaxxers who intentionally spread misinformation is really problematic.

No matter how you got COVID, or what your life is like, we need to maintain respect for one another. Much of the inherent power of patient-led or community-led movements in health conditions is that we're crossing over lines of difference in race, class, disability—and those differences have affected our risk of COVID infection and experiences with Long COVID. When we cross these lines and start demanding solidarity and real equity, then we have more power to recognize and fight for a lot of things that need to change.

Survival Tips

I. Remember that you are not alone. We are stronger together! Find community and support for yourself; whenever possible, contribute to support for others with Long COVID, and other chronically ill and disabled people, as you are able. Even if you only share that you are struggling, that opens up space for others to share that they are struggling, too.

2. Realize that the struggles you are facing and the barriers you encounter are likely not unique—they are probably systemic issues others are also facing. You can learn from what other people have encountered, find ways to support one another, and fight together to change these conditions—and you can win!

3. Check out organized groups and networks of people with Long COVID, and broader groups of chronically ill and disabled people, and join them. Groups with accountable leadership—where there are clearly-identified leaders, defined members, and ways for members to give input and also become leaders—can help us turn our individual challenges into collective campaigns for change and relief.

4. If you are a person of privilege—because of your economic or social class, formal education, race, gender, or positional power—consider how you can leverage that privilege to open doors for others, and how you can move back.

5. Be consistent in demanding that the full needs of people living with Long COVID are seen, documented, measured, centered, and resourced. And always remember that we're neither failures for being sick nor guilty or to blame for getting a health condition. As some people with Long COVID recover or respond to treatments, we must be vigilant about supporting one another no matter what our trajectory is, and not fall into ableist traps of blaming and shaming.

6. When in doubt, consider three guiding principles that have informed our work:

- We are not alone. Networks and community support have been crucial, both for our personal well-being and survival as chronically ill and disabled people and in our politics and collaborative efforts.

- We know what we need to survive and thrive. We have an individual and collective right to medical care, to support, and to resources. While professionals can help inform our options, we are best able to identify our priorities and what will most help us get through our challenges. Our knowledge is literally embodied as chronically ill and disabled people.

- Those who are most directly impacted—not just by our health conditions themselves but also by the broader political and economic circumstances that affect our risks and experiences of disease and disability that are shaped by gender, race, class, and other factors—**must be centered** in our groups, in our decision-making, and by those in positions of power over the systems we need to survive.

The Future of Long COVID

Learning from Patients & What Comes Next

Akiko Iwasaki, PhD

In the summer of 2020, I first learned about people suffering a variety of symptoms that last for much longer than expected following an acute respiratory infection. As an immunologist and researcher, I was more focused on trying to understand acute COVID in hospitalized patients in this early phase of the pandemic. At the time, we knew almost nothing about this disease, and our immediate concern was COVID deaths and hospitalizations. It wasn't until I received a phone call from journalist Ed Yong from *The Atlantic*, asking me to provide my take on why some people were experiencing long-term symptoms—what was being referred to as "Long COVID"—that I paid much attention to the longer consequences of SARS-CoV-2 infection.

That phone call changed my life. Since then, we have learned that, in Long COVID, acute COVID symptoms are compounded or replaced by overwhelming fatigue, shortness of breath, and neurological dysfunction, among over two hundred other symptoms that impact every organ imaginable. These long-term symptoms were occurring in many people with mild or asymptomatic infections—not just those with severe symptoms. After hearing from hundreds of long-haulers and learning more and more about the condition, I felt compelled to do something.

As an immunologist who has studied the basic mechanisms of infectious diseases caused by a number of viruses, I have decided to dive into research, with the goal of understanding the pathobiology of Long COVID. Infectious diseases develop through a combination of damage caused by the pathogen and the host's immune responses to the infection. Long COVID must also have varying degrees of involvement of the host and pathogen, but this may vary from person to person. In some, Long COVID may be driven mostly by the virus persisting in their organs, while others may develop autoimmunity. These events may occur in sequence in some and simultaneously in others.

Once I began to investigate the underlying mechanisms of Long COVID, the first person I reached out to was Dr. David Putrino, at the Mount Sinai School of Medicine, who sees and provides therapy to Long COVID patients and was already becoming a leading voice for Long COVID. *The worst that can happen is that he ignores my email,* I thought to myself. Fortunately, he responded immediately with a yes to collaboration. Since then, we have been working closely together to determine the immune profiles of long-haulers.

Now, we know a lot more about Long COVID. Studies have shown that Long COVID develops in approximately 50 percent of hospitalized COVID survivors and approximately 30 percent of nonhospitalized patients.[1] Women are at a higher risk of developing Long COVID than men.[2] Our work is revealing that distinct immune and physiological changes distinguish long-haulers from those who recover from acute COVID. For example, we see elevation in T cell exhaustion (which happens when T cells encounter persistent antigen), abnormal T cell cytokine profiles (set of cytokines that don't belong to typical antiviral responses), and increased activation of B cells (cells that secrete antibodies), among many other biological alterations. Some of these features are associated with distinct symptoms and differ between men and women. We are committed to developing more insights into the root causes of this disease.

The Long COVID Survival Guide is a collection of voices of people who have lived with Long COVID—honest, sincere, and at times gut-wrenching. Reading through the book, I had to take breaks multiple times to calm my sorrow and anger. Their suffering is immense and goes far beyond the physical pain. It involves social, mental, and financial struggles, as a quarter of long-haulers cannot return to work.[3] The voices in this book tell a story of a protracted battle against this debilitating condition—but also a story of finding inner strength and community. Learning to be okay with new conditions and asking for help is key to survival. Knowing that you are not the only one suffering in isolation—but are actually one of many millions around the world with similar health problems—provides a small but much-needed relief. As Alison Sbrana says in chapter 4, "This is not your fault."

This book reminds us of the efforts of patient-leaders who first raised awareness about Long COVID at the start of the pandemic and who originated the name for this condition. Since those early days, other terms, such as "post-acute sequelae of SARS-CoV-2 infection" (PASC) and "post-acute COVID-19 Syndrome" (PACS), have been coined by medical organizations seeking to describe it, but Long COVID is the term preferred by patients.

The Long COVID Survival Guide is also full of practical information; it's a how-to guide for people with Long COVID and those who take care of them. What can you expect from getting Long COVID? Common symptoms include postural orthostatic tachycardia syndrome (POTS) and dysautonomia (defined and explained well in chapter 2). Cognitive dysfunction (see chapter 8) and mental health issues (see chapter 7) are also experienced by most long-haulers, and this book provides helpful resources on those issues as well. There are also less widely discussed symptoms, like painful and prolonged menstrual bleeding (highlighted in chapter 9). The challenges of living with Long COVID can be immense, and it often takes more than one person to help you get through it. Chimére L. Smith recommends building a "care team" in chapter 5. The book is filled with crucial suggestions like Chimére's—from how and why you need to obtain a Long COVID diagnosis (see chapter 6) to how to get your medical bills covered by your health insurance or receive worker's compensation (see chapter 4).

Thanks to the efforts of patient advocates, in October 2021, Long COVID received an ICD-10 code, which can be used by physicians to bill insurance companies for appointments, testing, services rendered, and, one day, treatments. I watched this unfold; Long COVID went from being mostly ignored to being more widely recognized, thanks to the efforts of patient-leaders organizing and speaking out. And now that we have an ICD-10 code, medical records can be more easily mined for data on those with Long COVID, which can help scientists analyze risk factors, demographic features and underlying conditions associated with this disease, as well as what medicines and treatments are helpful or harmful.

However, getting a Long COVID diagnosis is not easy. This is, in part, due to the fact that we don't yet have a universal clinical definition of Long COVID and, in part, due to ignorance by health care providers. What questions do you ask to ensure that providers give you an accurate diagnosis and do not simply gaslight and dismiss you? I highly recommend arming yourself with a copy of these questions, provided by Dr. Putrino in chapter 6, at your appointments with health care providers:

1. "What is your differential diagnosis for my condition?"
2. "What is the evidence for and against that differential?"
3. "How have you ruled these differential diagnoses out?"
4. "Could you please document that?"

Asking for a differential diagnosis will encourage the provider to engage in both a deeper thought process and investigation into your symptoms.

Dr. Putrino's questions can help empower patients as they navigate health care systems. But where do you find research on Long COVID, and how do you go about interpreting the results? In chapter 11, Lisa McCorkell, cofounder of Patient-Led Research Collaborative, takes you through navigating the research world to understand how a study is designed and conducted and whether it is credible. Knowledge is power. Even if science hasn't figured out the precise mechanism of Long COVID, knowing what we don't know is sometimes just as powerful.

I personally benefited so much by reading early research from the Patient-Led Research Collaborative that described the duration, severity, and frequencies of various symptoms in different demographics.[4] Their findings were incredibly informative, as I was trying to grasp the breadth of symptoms and organ involvement as well as the duration of these symptoms. I have also learned and benefited from other reports written by patient groups, such as the impact of vaccination in long haulers,[5] leading to collaborative research with the Patient-Led Research Collaborative and Survivor Corps, a Facebook support group, to start to address the impact of vaccines on the immune profiles of people with Long COVID.[6] We rely on patients' experience and knowledge to guide research.

A common and deep frustration experienced by almost all the long-haulers in this book is that of being dismissed, or not believed, by health care providers. Being a woman, Latinx, Indigenous, Black, Asian, larger-bodied, a person of limited financial means, or an immigrant adds layers to this struggle, as medical professionals have dismissed the voices of these populations as "hysteria" for decades. It is outrageous that patients' suffering is dismissed because of ignorance and that these people who are desperately seeking help are seen through a biased lens. As an Asian immigrant woman, I understand how it feels to be treated differently because of the way I look. Such discrimination has no place in medicine or research; it drives me even more to get to the root cause of this disease, to help stop this ongoing gaslighting and discrimination.

Educating health care providers and cultivating humility and compassion in the medical profession are top priorities in the fight against Long COVID. Of course, more research and a better understanding of Long COVID and other post-acute infection syndromes (PAIS) will aid in providing much-needed evidence-based educational materials that can help providers understand the disease and provide patients with suitable treatment. Unfortunately, it seems that the lack of knowledge about PAIS starts in medical schools, where students rarely receive information on infection-initiated illnesses like ME/CFS. But every medical school should include a discussion of PAIS in their curriculum. These illnesses are becoming more common and can seemingly affect anyone.

One of the biggest surprises of Long COVID is that many people went from the height of productive careers and active lifestyles to being disabled almost overnight. Dreams have been dashed by this disease, and lives have been altered. In their introduction, Fiona Lowenstein sums up the reality of this disease: "I am not the person I was before I developed Long COVID, and I doubt I will ever feel I've returned to that former self, even if all of my remaining health issues someday evaporate." Countless other Long COVID survivors feel this way. It can take time to adjust to the reality of much-needed rest and pacing that Pato Hebert outlines in chapter 3.

Finally, this book is also about hope. Through much struggle, long-haulers find comfort in knowing others with similar symptoms. Finding peer-to-peer support is so important to surviving your Long COVID journey (see chapter 10). Patients are the experts of this disease, and they devote their time and effort in sharing their experiences, forming support groups everywhere. Long-haulers with backgrounds in science and medicine are conducting and publishing their own research, and the community relies on groups like the Patient-Led Research Collaborative to provide their latest research on Long COVID. In addition to our collaborative work with Dr. Putrino and Dr. Harlan Krumholz at Yale, we have launched an investigation of Long COVID symptoms and immune profiles through the Yale LISTEN study (Listen to Immune, System and Treatment Experiences Now), which seeks to understand Long COVID symptoms and immune responses by collecting information about symptoms and medical history from members of patient communities.[7] We are also enrolling participants who experience chronic symptoms after vaccination. Research gives us insights and hope for understanding the disease and developing effective therapies.

Prolonged illness from infection is not unique to Long COVID. A number of other infections—the pandemic flu, dengue, polio, SARS, Ebola virus, West Nile virus, Epstein-Barr virus, as well as the bacterial infections that cause Lyme disease (*Borrelia burgdorferi*) and Q fever (after *Coxiella burnetii* infection)—are known to cause debilitating prolonged symptoms that lead to ME/CFS. But, because of the sheer number of people infected by SARS-CoV-2 around the globe, Long COVID has become overwhelming and must not be dismissed. Prior to the COVID pandemic, about 2.5 million Americans were already living with ME/CFS (see chapter 4). With a percentage of Long COVID patients developing ME/CFS, that number is expected to grow significantly. A wealth of information built by patients with ME/CFS provides an invaluable resource to those who are entering the world of PAIS for the first time (see chapter 12).[8]

I am so grateful to the authors of this book for providing a real-world account of living through the various phases of PAIS, which should provide a lesson for the future. There is a dire need for research: patient-facing research to help with symptoms to help patients get through their daily lives a bit easier as well as pathogenesis-facing research to get at the root cause of this disease, so we can better design clinical trials to find treatments that directly benefit patients. When the next pandemic arrives, my hope is that we will be better able to deal with PAIS from all possible angles: prevention, diagnosis, treatment, and medical care, as well as financial, social, mental, and global support of those who suffer from PAIS. Long COVID has changed the narrative. The world no longer has any excuse to make the same mistake over and over again, as we have done for previous pandemic and endemic infections. It's finally time for us to listen.

Akiko Iwasaki (she/her) is a Sterling Professor of Immunobiology at the Yale University School of Medicine. She received her PhD in immunology from the University of Toronto (1998) and completed her postdoctoral training at the National Institutes of Health before joining Yale's faculty in 2000. Dr. Iwasaki has been a Howard Hughes Medical Institute Investigator since 2014. Her research focuses on immune responses to viral infections and infectious disease mechanisms. Her team has developed new approaches to vaccines, such as Prime and Pull and Prime and Spike. She was elected to the National Academy of Sciences in 2018, the National Academy of Medicine in 2019, the American Academy of Microbiology in 2020, and the American Academy of Arts and Sciences in 2021. Dr. Iwasaki is at the forefront of COVID-19 pandemic, with respect to research, science communication, and public service. She is also well known for her advocacy on women and underrepresented minorities in the science and medicine fields and has a large follower base on social media. She is the director of a newly built Yale Center for Infection and Immunity, where she leads groups of investigators to study infectious origin of many chronic diseases, including Long COVID.

Glossary

These definitions were collectively compiled by our contributors, who drew from the knowledge in their chapters, the WHO and CDC websites, the National Alliance on Mental Illness, and #MEAction's ME-pedia, among other sources. Some of these terms have multiple meanings. We have done our best to convey nuance when possible.

Ableism: typically refers to a system of oppression that disadvantages and/ or discriminates against disabled people. Disability justice activist Mia Mingus has said that "ableism is connected to all our struggles because it undergirds notions of whose bodies are considered valuable, desirable and disposable."

"Backpay" (for Social Security, both SSDI and SSI): because it can take a long time to be approved for these programs, "backpay" compensates people for the benefit amount they should have been receiving while waiting for approval of their application. There are some complexities that affect backpay—the date of an application, the date the disability began, a 5-month waiting period for SSDI, lawyer fees paid on contingency that are paid from backpay, as well as the type of program you are applying for (SSDI vs. SSI).

Acute COVID: a term long-haulers and researchers sometimes use to try to differentiate between the immediate phase of illness, which often follows an initial infection, and Long COVID symptoms, winch may persist or develop over time.

Aging and Disability Resource Center (ADRC): government offices that help people understand options for long term services and supports. This can be support such as help at home with tasks like showering safely, getting dressed (including compression stockings for those with POTS), medication management, meal preparation, doing laundry, maintaining air filters or humidifiers, light housework, getting around your home and community safely, help with physical therapy, and other tasks based on the individual's need and the support service options.

Akathisia: a movement disorder that can make it hard to stay still.

Americans with Disabilities Act (ADA): the ADA is the 1990 civil rights law protecting people with disabilities from discrimination and giving them equal opportunity to participate in life activities, including employment.

Antibody tests: a blood test that's done to detect whether a person has been previously infected with SARS-CoV-2, the virus that causes COVID-19. Nuclear antibodies corroborate infection in the months that follow acute COVID (and offer a sense of when the acute infection may have occurred). But not all Long COVID patients produce these antibodies, so these tests cannot be used to rule out a COVID-19 infection. In fact, the absence of antibodies may also be an indicator of Long COVID. Surface antibodies alone suggest a response to vaccination, as vaccines have been developed from surface antigens of SARS-CoV-2.

Antinuclear antibodies (ANA): a blood test that measures the amount and pattern of antibodies in your blood that work against your own body.

Antiviral treatments: medicines that are designed to assist the body in clearing or quelling lingering or reactivated viral infections that are causing symptoms (e.g., taking acyclovir for a herpes simplex/cold sore outbreak).

Assisted suicide: suicide undertaken with the aid of another person, often facilitated by a family member and/or physician at the wish of someone with a terminal illness.

Autoantibodies: a blood protein (antibody) that is produced by the body and designed to react to the body's own tissues. This is unusual because antibodies typically react to foreign substances, not parts of our own body.

Autoimmune disease/ autoimmunity: occurs when the immune system mistakenly attacks the body instead of protecting it. One of the common triggers of autoimmune disease is infection.

Autonomic nervous system: the part of the human nervous system that does a lot of things in the background "autonomously" (i.e., without asking us for conscious permission to do so) to keep our body functioning. Composed of the sympathetic and parasympathetic nervous systems.

Basic metabolic panel: a common blood test that measures eight different substances in your blood, providing helpful information about a body's chemical balance and metabolism.

Beta-blockers: a class of medications that block the activation of a specific type of receptor on the heart, resulting in reduced cardiac action. As such, beta blockers can help to reduce heart rate and blood pressure.

Biomarkers: a broad category of medical signs that indicate a normal or abnormal process, or of the presence of a condition or disease.

Bipolar disorder: a mental illness that causes dramatic shifts in a person's mood, energy and ability to think clearly. People with bipolar disorder experience high and low moods, known as mania and depression.

Bradycardia: slower-than-expected heart rate, generally beating fewer than 60 beats per minute.

Brain fog: a colloquial term for cognitive dysfunction, often characterized by issues with memory, focus, verbal communication, visual and auditory processing, problem solving, and/or motor-functioning.

Cellular level medicine: also referred to as *cellular medicine*, a branch of medicine that attempts to link abnormal biological function to dysfunction at the cellular level, with a focus on interventions that specifically affect cellular functioning.

Centers for Independent Living (CIL): US community-based nonprofits run by people with disabilities to help people with disabilities. To find a location near you, go to the Administration for Community Living website at ACL.gov.

Chest X-ray: an imaging test that uses X-rays to look at the structures and organs in the chest, which enables a health care provider to see how well the lungs and heart are working.

Cognitive behavioral therapy (CBT): a type of psychological therapy that attempts to solve psychological problems by retraining ways of thinking and patterns of behavior. Historically, providers who believe chronic illnesses are psychological in origin have harmfully prescribed CBT to people with complex chronic illnesses as a *curative* treatment.

Cognitive therapy: a kind of brain injury rehabilitation program focused on improving areas of cognition, such as memory, attention, problem solving, organization, executive function skills, and word finding.

Co-infections: when multiple pathogens (i.e., bacterial or viral) are infecting the body simultaneously.

Comorbidity: a disease or medical condition that is simultaneously present in a patient who has another or other diseases or medical conditions.

Complete blood count: a set of common blood tests that provide information about the cells in a person's blood–such as counts of white blood cells, red blood cells, and platelets—the concentration of hemoglobin, and the hematocrit.

Complex post-traumatic stress disorder (C-PTSD): a condition that involves many of the same symptoms of PTSD, along with other psychiatric and cognitive symptoms. Often characterized by ongoing trauma.

Confounding variable: a factor that influences both variables that are being studied but is not being studied itself. For example, let's say a study finds that the more ice cream is consumed, the more sunburns occur. A confounding variable here is a heat wave. A heat wave would cause more ice cream to be consumed and more sunburns to occur. But if heat waves are not taken into account in the study design and analysis, someone might infer an incorrect causal relationship between ice cream and sunburns.

COVID-19 long-hauler: a term used to describe people with Long COVID, coined by Long COVID patient-advocate Amy Watson, as she waited for a PCR test while wearing a trucker-style cap.

Craniosacral therapy: an alternative therapy where a practitioner uses gentle, light touch to help address restrictions in fascia (connective tissue) to promote fluid movement in and around the nervous system and spine.

Crash: a colloquial term for a symptom flare or worsened health, often following exertion.

C-reactive protein (CRP): a blood test that measures the level of C-reactive protein, a protein made by the liver and sent into your bloodstream in response to inflammation.

Cytokine panels: blood tests that identify elevated levels of specific cytokines, used for understanding the pathophysiology of immune, infectious, inflammatory disorders and for research purposes.

Cytokines: a class of proteins that are involved in cell process signaling, they are typically very involved in initiating and maintaining immune reactions such as inflammation.

D-dimer: blood test that screens for blood clotting disorders.

Denver Principles: a kind of "Bill of Rights" for people living with HIV, created in 1983 at the fifth annual Gay and Lesbian Health Conference in Denver. The Denver Principles demanded the right to a voice in decision making on the HIV research, care, and treatment agenda; to be treated with full respect and dignity; and to be recognized as experts in their own right.

Diagnostic codes: a tool to group and identify diseases, disorders, symptoms, poisonings, adverse effects of drugs and chemicals, injuries and other reasons for patient encounters.

Differential diagnosis: a method of analysis of a patient's history and physical examination to arrive at the correct diagnosis.

Dysautonomia: a simple name for a complex group of medical conditions caused by dysregulation of the autonomic nervous system (ANS), the part of your nervous system that controls basically all the things your body does that you don't really think about or consciously make a decision to do: breathing, digestion, heart rate, blood pressure, body temperature, sleep cycles, bladder function, hormonal function, and more. Symptoms can include orthostatic (posture-related) intolerance, fatigue, shortness of breath, blurred vision, cognitive impairments, and fainting, among others.

Eczema: a form of inflammation of the skin that often has no obvious external cause but results in patches of the skin becoming rough, inflamed, and covered in blisters.

Ehlers-Danlos syndrome: EDS are a group of hereditary disorders of connective tissue that are varied in the ways they affect the body. They are generally characterized by joint hypermobility, joint instability, skin hyperextensibility, and other structural weaknesses.

Energy envelope: Energy Envelope Theory is a self-management tool developed and tested by Dr. Leonard Jason to reduce symptom severity and the frequency of relapses for people with ME/CFS. According to this theory, ME/CFS patients should not expend more energy than they perceive they have because doing so results in post-exertional malaise and higher disability. A person's "energy envelope" is typically the amount of energy a patient can expend, given the physical limits their disease may have imposed on them.

Epstein-Barr virus: one of the most common human viruses, found all over the world. Epstein-Barr virus (also referred to as EBV and human herpesvirus 4) is a member of the herpes virus family and can cause infectious mononucleosis, also known as *mono* in addition to other illnesses. Most people get infected with EBV at some point in their lives.

Erythrocyte sedimentation rate (ESR or sed rate): a blood test that measures how quickly erythrocytes (red blood cells) settle at the bottom of a test tube that contains a blood sample. Normally, red blood cells settle relatively slowly. A faster-than-normal rate may indicate inflammation in the body.

Extrapolating results: applies the results of a narrower study to a broader population.

#FBLC: a hashtag people with Long COVID use to connect with one another online. It stands for "Follow Back Long COVID."

Functional magnetic resonance imagining (fMRI): a technique for measuring and mapping brain activity by detecting changes associated with blood flow. While an MRI creates images of a patient's organs, tissue, or bones, an fMRI shows the function of the brain.

Functional medicine: a branch of medicine that focuses on working holistically with a patient in order to identify root causes for symptoms, rather than focusing on single-specialty symptomatic care that fails to address complex health issues with interconnected symptoms across specialty domains.

Generalized anxiety disorder: chronic feelings of intense worry, fear, and distress that can consume hours each day, making it hard to concentrate or finish routine daily tasks.

Gut dysbiosis: an imbalance of bacteria in the gut.

HELP-apheresis: a therapeutic technique that has been used for systemic conditions, such as certain cancers, autoimmune conditions, and cholesterol disorders. HELP-apheresis is a form of apheresis that is now being pioneered by Dr. Beate Jaeger, in Germany, for people with Long COVID. HELP-apheresis seems to reduce the presentation of microclots in the blood of people with Long COVID and has been associated with an improvement in their symptoms.

High-sensitivity C-reactive protein (hs-CRP): a blood test that is more sensitive than a standard CRP test and finds lower levels of C-reactive protein.

Histamines: chemicals in the immune system that react to perceived allergens, often by inducing sneezing, tearing up, or itchiness.

Holter monitor test: a twenty-four-hour electrocardiogram (ECG) that monitors one's heart rate by measuring the time between each beat. It is considered an accurate way of picking up on instances of bradycardia (slow heart rate) or tachycardia (fast heart rate).

Human herpesvirus 6 (HHV-6): a very common form of herpesvirus, that is typically present in most people from early life but can reactivate in later life to cause significant health problems.

Humoral response: The body's first line of defense to a foreign substance entering the body, consisting of the immune system producing cells, proteins and other inflammatory chemicals that attempt to protect the body from incoming invaders.

Hyperbaric oxygen therapy (HBOT): A form of therapy that allows users to be exposed to highly specific concentrations and pressures of oxygen for a limited period of time.

Hypermobility spectrum disorder: connective tissue disorders characterized by symptomatic joint hypermobility, such as any Ehlers-Danlos syndrome.

Infection-initiated illness: a typically chronic illness triggered by an infection.

Inflammation: a bodily reaction where chemicals that are produced by white blood cells enter the body's tissues to protect the body from foreign invaders or respond to tissue damage.

Insomnia: a sleep disorder characterized by trouble falling asleep and/or staying asleep.

Integrative medicine: a branch of medicine that integrates principles of both Western medicine as well as other branches of alternative medicine (such as traditional Chinese medicine) in order to treat illness.

International Classification of Diseases (ICD): a tool that assigns codes for diseases, symptoms, abnormal findings, and other circumstances.

Invisible disability: not all disabled people have visible physical disabilities; many Long COVID patients, in particular, may read as nondisabled to people who are not aware of their illness. This doesn't mean they are not disabled. The term *invisible disability* is often used to describe such situations.

Irritable bowel syndrome (IBS): a common gastrointestinal condition, often characterized by abdominal pain or discomfort.

Liver function tests: also referred to as hepatic panels, LFTs are blood tests that measure different enzymes, proteins, and other substances made by the liver to check the overall health of the liver.

Long COVID: COVID-19 long-hauler and advocate Elisa Perego coined the term, which refers to a range of infection-associated illnesses that present as new, returning, or ongoing health problems experienced by people four or more weeks after their initial coronavirus infection. Rarely, similar prolonged symptoms have been reported with SARS-CoV-2 vaccination.

Major depressive disorder: a mental illness defined by persistently depressed mood or loss of interest in activities that significantly impairs one's ability to function in daily life.

Mast cell activation syndrome (MCAS): a condition in which someone experiences chronic allergy symptoms or symptoms of anaphylaxis. Symptoms can include hives, swelling, low blood pressure, difficulty breathing, and gastrointestinal distress, among other issues.

ME/CFS: myalgic encephalomyelitis—once called chronic fatigue syndrome and often abbreviated as ME/CFS—is a complex chronic disease that presents with symptoms in multiple body systems. It is a neurological disease according to the World Health Organization, and its hallmark symptom is post-exertional malaise (PEM) or symptom exacerbation.

Meaningful involvement: popularized by the HIV/AIDS movement through the acronym MIPA (meaningful involvement of people with HIV/AIDS), the term calls for ensuring that the communities most affected by a medical condition are involved in decision-making, at every level of the response, not only as individuals but as representatives of organized groups.

Medicaid and Child Health Insurance Program (CHIP): Medicaid is run by each state (as opposed to Medicare, which is a federal program) and provides medical benefits to people with disabilities, people aged sixty-five and older, adults with low incomes, children, and pregnant women. CHIP is for kids up to age nineteen, and kids can qualify even when income is too high for Medicaid. These programs take applications at any time, as opposed to state health care marketplace plans, which limit open enrollment to specific periods of time.

Medical gaslighting: a term used to describe doctors or medical practitioners who blame a patient's illness or symptoms on psychological factors or deny a patient's illness entirely, the impact of which may result in the experience of invalidation and lack of further diagnostic workup/ treatment.

Medicare: a US federal health insurance program for people 65 years of age and older, as well as disabled individuals on Social Security Disability Income (SSDI) whose coverage starts two years after the disability date Social Security determines.

Methodology: the plan for how to conduct and analyze a study.

Microbiome: in human health, the term *microbiome* typically refers to a vast collection of different species of bacteria that coexist on our bodies, interacting with each other and our tissue to support daily bodily functions.

Microclots/microthrombi: small clots that are not large enough to block major blood vessels or cause life-threatening events but are large enough to affect the function of multiple organs. Microclots have been found in many people with Long COVID.

Microvascular damage: organ damage caused by reduced blood flow of small blood vessels.

Migraine: a severe and debilitating, often unilateral and pulsatile (marked by pulsations) headache disorder that is often preceded by signs and symptoms, or auras, such as visual or auditory disturbances or nausea.

#MillionsMissing: a campaign designed by ME/CFS advocacy organization #MEAction to recognize the millions of people who have been sidelined from society due to a lack of support for their chronic illnesses and/or disabilities. It also refers to the millions of dollars missing from clinical education and research on ME/CFS.

Mitochondrial dysfunction: a disruption in the ability of the body's cells to produce energy.

#NEISVoid: a hashtag started by disability advocate Brianne Bennes to connect a community that believes people first, refrains from unsolicited advice, and truly listens to the struggles of those with chronic illnesses. It stands for "No End in Sight Void."

Neuronal activity: how your brain functions to make and maintain neurological connections.

Neuroplasticity: the ability of the brain to form and reorganize synaptic connections, especially in response to learning or experience or following injury, much greater in youth but still present in adults.

Orthostatic intolerance: the inability to be upright without feeling dizziness, lightheadedness, vertigo, or increased heart rate, among other symptoms. Often a defining symptom associated with POTS and/or dysautonomia.

Oxidative stress: changes to the chemical balance of cells that can cause damage.

Pacing: a self-management strategy and technique for managing symptoms and exertion—especially helpful for people experiencing post-exertional malaise (PEM) symptom exacerbation. Chronically ill people who pace well are active when able and rest when tired. Often, people practicing pacing may plan extra rest ahead of and after planned periods of exertion.

Parasympathetic nervous system: works in tandem with the sympathetic nervous system. Once our bodies decide a threat has passed, our parasympathetic nervous system kicks in to return our body to homeostasis, bringing our breathing back to normal, lowering our blood pressure and heart rate, returning our hormones to their normal levels, and allowing us to get back to the "rest and digest" state.

Pathogen: disease-causing agent (bacteria, virus, parasite, etc.).

Pathogenesis: how a disease or injury starts and develops over time in the body.

Pathophysiology: the processes occurring in the body that result in disease or injury.

PCR test: polymerase chain reaction test, which is one way of achieving a molecular diagnosis for acute COVID. A PCR test can detect the presence of viral RNA for up to approximately twenty days. It is thought to be most sensitive during a short window of time at the beginning of a COVID infection, and for this and other reasons, up to 25 percent of PCR tests and 50 percent of rapid antigen tests result in false negatives. Many COVID long-haulers do not have positive PCR test results confirming their infections, due to accessibility and test reliability issues.

Peer-reviewed article: a scientific paper that has gone through an evaluation process by experts in the field.

Perimenopause: the period of time during which a menstruating person's body makes the transition to menopause.

Personal protective equipment (PPE): according to the United States Department of Labor Occupational Safety and Health Administration, PPE is equipment worn to minimize exposure to hazards that cause serious workplace injuries and illnesses. Throughout the pandemic, and especially at the start, there have been supply issues that have resulted in health care workers needing to reuse PPE or not being able to access it at all.

Post-acute sequelae of SARS-CoV-2 (PASC): the current term the National Institutes of Health uses for "Long COVID."

Post-concussion syndrome (PCS): when concussion symptoms persist for months or years after a traumatic brain injury or other type of brain trauma.

Post-exertional malaise/post-exertional symptom exacerbation: the worsening of symptoms or the development of new symptoms following mental, physical, or emotional exertion. A common symptom experienced by people with ME/CFS and Long COVID, as well as related conditions. Often abbreviated as "PEM" online and in support groups. PEM is a hallmark symptom of ME/CFS and is also common for COVID long-haulers.

Post-traumatic stress disorder (PTSD): a disorder characterized by long-term symptoms following a traumatic event that may include intrusive and distressing memories, avoidance, and/or hypervigilance, among other symptoms.

Postural orthostatic tachycardia syndrome (POTS): a form of dysautonomia that occurs when the autonomic nervous system has trouble regulating heart rate.

Post-viral illness: an illness triggered by viral infection, typically chronic.

Preexisting condition: often used in reference to health insurance, a pre-existing condition is an existing health problem a person had before that person's health insurance went into effect or before that person contracted another condition. Prior to 2014, in the United States, some health insurance companies were allowed to exclude patients with pre-existing conditions from coverage.

Premenstrual dysphoric disorder (PMDD): a severe form of premenstrual syndrome that includes physical and behavioral symptoms—including extreme mood shifts that can disrupt work and relationships—that usually subside or stop with the onset of menstruation.

Pre-print: an earlier version of a scientific paper that is posted online before it goes through a formal peer review process.

Psychosis: characterized as disruptions to a person's thoughts and perceptions that make it difficult for them to recognize what is real and what isn't.

Pulse oximeter: a device that can estimate the oxygen saturation of the blood and pulse rate, usually worn on the finger. A pulse oximeter can be helpful for monitoring your health at home.

#pwLC: a hashtag people with Long COVID use to connect with one another online. It stands for "people with Long COVID."

#pwME: a hashtag people with ME/CFS use to connect with one another online. It stands for "people with ME."

Rapid antigen test: similar to a PCR test, rapid antigen tests can detect the shedding of viral proteins. They are most sensitive during a short time window at the beginning of a COVID infection, and for this and other reasons, up to 50 percent of rapid antigen tests result in false negatives.

Relapsing-remitting or episodic illness: a typically chronic illness with symptoms that wax and wane, often characterized by post-exertional symptom exacerbation and/or crashes.

Screen sensitivity: symptom exacerbation from using screens, such as phones and laptops.

Secondary infections: infections that occur after an immediately preceding infection creates vulnerability (often these are secondary bacterial infections following primary viral infections).

Sequelae: a condition or symptoms that are the consequence of a prior disease or injury.

Seroconversion: a term that describes the body's change from a seronegative to seropositive state. In the context of COVID-19, it refers to individuals who transition from a state of not producing antibodies for the COVID-19 virus to producing antibodies as a result of COVID-19 infection or vaccination.

Severe acute respiratory syndrome (SARS): a viral respiratory disease caused by a SARS-associated coronavirus, first identified in 2003 during an outbreak that emerged in China and spread to four other countries.

Short- and long-term disability insurance: in the US, this type of disability benefit is typically accessed through your employer, although individuals can get their own policies. This benefit helps pay a portion of your income if you are not able to work due to illness or disability. You only have access to this if you had coverage through your employer or if you have your own individual plan; it's not a government benefit. Specific policies vary. Sometimes referred to as private disability insurance and sometimes abbreviated in support groups as "STD" and "LTD."

Small fiber neuropathy (SFN): a disorder that occurs when the small fibers of the peripheral nervous system are damaged; can cause sensory symptoms, including pain, burning, and tingling.

Social determinants of health: the conditions in the variety of environments in which people live that impact health outcomes.

Social Security Disability Insurance (SSDI): in the US, a disability benefit through Social Security for workers who have enough work credits with Social Security. SSDI differs from Supplemental Security Income (SSI). To find out if you have enough work credits to apply for SSDI, make an account on the Social Security website, SSA.gov, where it will show you your estimated monthly amount if you were to become disabled today. You may be eligible to apply based on

your spouse or parent's Social Security, depending on various factors. Recipients get Medicare coverage after two years. The definition of disability is based on if your condition is expected to last for at least a year, if you are able to work at a certain level (called substantial gainful activity), and if your medical condition is severe or on their list of medical conditions. There is no asset test for SSDI, which means they will not consider your household's income when determining benefits. If you are eligible, you can work part-time under a certain level while receiving benefits. Monthly benefits are calculated based on your work history; in January 2022, average monthly benefits were $1,358.50.

Somatoform disorders: somatization, which stems from a history of the hysteria diagnosis used to explain (away) illnesses in mostly women, is the belief that emotional distress turns into physical symptoms. Somatoform disorders are typically diagnosed based on symptoms, rather than testing criteria.

Spoon theory/spoons/spoonies: a metaphor that uses spoons as visual tools to conceptualize units of mental or physical energy available for daily activities and tasks, developed by Christine Miserandino. Spoon theory is a helpful tool for chronically ill people to plan what we will spend our limited energy on and generally involves interspersing energy-draining activities with periods of rest. Chronically ill and/or disabled people who ascribe to spoon theory sometimes refer to ourselves and one another as "spoonies" and refer to our energy as "spoons."

Statistically significant: occurs when a finding is not likely to have occurred by chance but, importantly, does not necessarily mean clinically significant.

Stem cell therapy: regenerative medicine that guides master cells to produce specialized cells that may have been lost or injured.

Superbill: a detailed invoice outlining the services received, which you can submit to your insurance if a provider doesn't correspond with insurance companies directly.

Supine: lying face upward, a position that helps ease symptoms for patients with POTS or other types of dysautonomia.

Supplemental Security Income (SSI): administered by Social Security in the US, this program is not the same as Social Security benefits that older adults receive and is also different from Social Security Disability Insurance (SSDI), the program that disabled people with enough Social Security work credits can access. This program is for people with disabilities or people sixty-five and older with very little to no income or resources. There is an asset test for your household, which is extremely low; as of January 2022, the limit is $2,000 total for an individual or child and $3,000 total for a couple. This limit includes cash, bank accounts, stocks, mutual funds, as well as things like vehicles and personal property or money given from friends or family. You can apply if you don't have enough work credits for SSDI. Working while receiving SSI affects your benefit amount, but there are rules and programs to help address this. The monthly benefit in 2022 was $841 per month for an individual; some states supplement this amount.

Sympathetic nervous system: primarily responsible for the body's fight-or-flight response; it's the thing that revs up when it senses stress or danger, sending out a flood of hormones to boost the body's alertness and heart rate, making sure your muscles have enough blood, your brain has enough oxygen, and your blood has enough glucose to handle whatever threat it deems imminent.

Tachycardia: a rapid heartbeat that may be regular or irregular but is out of proportion to age and level of exertion or activity.

T-cell: a type of white blood cell that helps to mediate the initial immune reaction to a foreign substance that enters the body.

Telehealth: health care accessed via virtual methods, often via a video call.

Temperature sensitivity: an excessive physiological or behavioral response to a change in temperature, which may result in heat or cold intolerance.

Temporary Assistance for Needy Families (TANF): monthly cash assistance to low-income families with children. Programs vary by state, and the name of the program may be different also.

Thyroid function tests: blood tests used to check the function of the thyroid.

Tilt table test: one way of diagnosing POTS. During a tilt table test, a patient lies on a table that raises their body from horizontal to vertical, to mimic standing straight up, and measures their heart rate and blood pressure. Patients often faint, even if they have never fainted before, because they can't call upon the physical coping mechanisms they've put into place over the years, like sitting or lying down, crossing their legs or fidgeting. Patients often report intense fatigue for a few days after the test, but an IV of saline solution can sometimes mitigate the onset of malaise. If a patient's symptoms are in line with standard dysautonomia symptoms, and other conditions have been ruled out, a doctor might opt for a "poor man's tilt table test" in their office. During these tests, patients go from a lying position to a sitting position and a sitting position to a standing position while wearing a simple pulse oximeter on their finger.

Tinnitus: ringing noises in one or both ears, typically not caused by an external sound.

Unemployment insurance benefits: benefits to support people who have lost their job and are looking for a new job. In the US, the Department of Labor administers these benefits in partnership with each state, so programs vary by state. Specific eligibility criteria vary, but typically you must be willing and able to work as well as actively looking for work, which contradicts disability determination for benefits (unable to work).

Vagus nerve stimulation (VNS): electrical stimulation of a nerve in your neck that is approved in treatment-resistant epilepsy, depression, and stroke.

Variable: a factor that is subject to change.

Vascular disease: diseases of the blood vessels that reduces blood flow to organs.

Vasovagal syncope: a sudden drop in heart rate and blood pressure, often leading to fainting, and often in reaction to a trigger.

Viral persistence: from Epstein-Barr to Zika virus, there's a rich body of literature to suggest that, in many cases of viral infection, a virus can continue to live in different tissues of the human body for years after the initial acute infection. Some researchers believe viral persistence may be a root cause of Long COVID.

Workers' compensation: workers who are injured or get sick as a result of their job are protected by these laws, and employers pay for insurance coverage for it. Benefits typically provide medical expense coverage and help with replacing income during recovery. Laws and benefits vary by location.

Notes

INTRODUCTION: ALL YOU NEED IS ONE PERSON

1. "Post-COVID Conditions," Centers for Disease Control, last modified September 16, 2021, https://www.cdc.gov/coronavirus/2019-ncov/long-term-effects/index.html.

CHAPTER 1: IT WASN'T THE BEANS AND RICE

1. Paige Nong et al., "Patient-Reported Experiences of Discrimination in the US Health Care System," *JAMA Network Open* 3, no. 12 (2020).

2. "Risk for COVID-19 Infection, Hospitalization, and Death By Race/Ethnicity," Centers for Disease Control, last modified March 25, 2022, https://www.cdc.gov/coronavirus/2019-ncov/covid-data/investigations-discovery/hospitalization-death-by-race-ethnicity.html.

3. Anthony P. Carnevale et al., "The Unequal Race for Good Jobs: How Whites Made Outsized Gains in Education and Good Jobs Compared to Blacks and Latinos," Georgetown University Center on Education and the Workforce, accessed April 13, 2022, https://cew.georgetown.edu/wp-content/uploads/ES-The_Unequal_Race_for_Good_Jobs.pdf; "Labor Force Statistics from the Current Population Survey," U.S. Bureau of Labor Statistics, last modified January 20, 2022, https://www.bls.gov/cps/cpsaat11.htm.

4. Daniel Cox et al., "Race, Religion, and Political Affiliation of Americans' Core Social Networks," *PRRI*, August 3, 2016.

5. Ariana Case et al., "Hispanic and Latino Representation in Film: Erasure On Screen & Behind the Camera Across 1,300 Popular Movies," USC Annenberg Inclusion Initiative, accessed April 14, 2022, https://assets.uscannenberg.org/docs/aii-hispanic-latino-rep-2021-09-13.pdf.

6. Luis Noe-Bustamante et al., "For U.S. Latinos, COVID-19 Has Taken a Personal and Financial Toll," Pew Research Center, July 15, 2021.

7. bell hooks, *All About Love: New Visions* (New York: William Morrow, 2018).

CHAPTER 2: STANDING TALL (AND SITTING RIGHT BACK DOWN)

1. "Dysautonomia," Cleveland Clinic, last modified July 10, 2020, my.clevelandclinic.org/health/diseases/6004-dysautonomia.

2. "Dysautonomia International," Dysautonomia International, accessed April 13, 2022, http://www.dysautonomiainternational.org.

3. "Summary of Syncopal Disorders," Dysautonomia International, accessed April 14, 2022, http://www.dysautonomiainternational.org/page.php?ID=31.

4. "Postural Orthostatic Tachycardia Syndrome," Dysautonomia International, accessed April 14, 2022, http://www.dysautonomiainternational.org/page.php?ID=30.

5. David Cox, "Why are Women More Prone to Long Covid?," *The Guardian*, June 13, 2021.

6. Jennifer Brea, *What Happens When You Have a Disease Doctors Can't Diagnose*, filmed June 2016 in Banff, Alberta, video, 16:59, https://www.ted.com/talks/jennifer_brea_what_happens_when_you_have_a_disease_doctors_can_t_diagnose?language=en.

7. Judith H. Lichtman et al., "Symptom Recognition and Healthcare Experiences of Young Women with Acute Myocardial Infarction," *Cardiovascular Quality and Outcomes* 8 (2015): S31–38.

8. Gabrielle Rosina Chiaramonte, "Physicians' Gender Bias in the Diagnosis, Treatment, and Interpretation of Coronary Heart Disease Symptoms," PhD diss., Stony Brook University, 2007, https://dspace.sunyconnect.suny.edu/bitstream/handle/1951/44285.

9. Maya Dusenbery, "Is Medicine's Gender Bias Killing Young Women?," *Pacific Standard*, February 7, 2018.

CHAPTER 3: COVID CAN'T BE OUTPACED

1. "Spoon Theory," Wikipedia, last modified April 14, 2022, https://en.wikipedia.org/wiki/Spoon_theory#.

2. "Post-exertional malaise," MEpedia, last modified April 14, 2022, https://me-pedia.org/wiki/Post-exertional_malaise.

3. *Merriam-Webster*, "stop, v.," accessed April 14, 2022, https://www.merriam-webster.com/dictionary/stop.

4. *Merriam-Webster*, "rest, n.," accessed April 14, 2022, https://www.merriam-webster.com/dictionary/rest.

5. *Merriam-Webster*, "pace, n.," accessed April 14, 2022, https://www.merriam-webster.com/dictionary/pace.

6. Maanvi Singh, "California's First Surgeon General on Covid: 'Greatest Collective Trauma' of a Generation," *The Guardian*, February 19, 2022.

CHAPTER 4: WITH DISABILITY, COMES RIGHTS

1. "Calculations & Formulas," COVID-19 Longhauler Advocacy Project, accessed April 14, 2022, https://www.longhauler-advocacy.org/calculations-formulas.

2. "What Is ME/CFS?," Center for Disease Control, last modified January 27, 2021, https://www.cdc.gov/me-cfs/about/index.html.

3. "MS Prevalence," National Multiple Sclerosis Society, accessed April 14, 2022, https://www.nationalmssociety.org/About-the-Society/MS-Prevalence.

4. "What Does #NEISVoid Mean?," No End in Sight, accessed April 14, 2022, https://noendinsight.co/neisvoid-explained.

5. "Monthly Statistical Snapshot,", Social Security Administration, accessed April 14, 2022, https://www.ssa.gov/policy/docs/quickfacts/stat_snapshot.

6. Ibid.

7. "Resources: For Providers," Body Politic, accessed April 14, 2022, https://www.wearebodypolitic.com/resources-for-providers.

CHAPTER 6: THE OBSTACLE COURSE

1. "What Is Somatic Symptom Disorder?," American Psychiatric Association, accessed April 13, 2022, https://www.psychiatry.org/patients-families/somatic-symptom-disorder/what-is-somatic-symptom-disorder.

2. "Job Accommodation Network," Job Accommodation Network, accessed April 13, 2022, https://askjan.org.

3. "Hyperbaric oxygen therapy," MEpedia, last modified March 19, 2021, https://me-pedia.org/wiki/Hyperbaric_oxygen_therapy.

4. Hannah Balfour, "Long-COVID symptoms improved with neuromodulation," *European Pharmaceutical Review*, July 9, 2021.

5. Greg Maguire, "Stem Cells Part of the Innate and Adaptive Immune Systems as a Therapeutic for Covid-19," *Communicative & Integrative Biology* 14, no. 1 (2021): 186–98.

6. Jon Hamilton, "From Blood Clots to Infected Neurons, How COVID Threatens the Brain," *NPR*, December 16, 2021.

7. "Long COVID Linked to Unbalanced Gut Microbiome: What to Know Now," *Healthline*, accessed April 13, 2022, https://www.healthline.com/health-news/long-covid-linked-to-unbalanced-gut-microbiome-what-to-know-now#Exact-cause-of-long-COVID-unknown.

8. "COVID-19 (coronavirus): Long-term effects," Mayo Clinic, last modified October 22, 2021, https://www.mayoclinic.org/diseases-conditions/coronavirus/in-depth/coronavirus-long-term-effects/art-20490351#.

9. Hasan K. Siddiqi et al., "COVID-19—A Vascular Disease," *Trends Cardiovasc Med.* 31, no. 1 (2021): 1–5, https://doi.org/10.1016/j.tcm.2020.10.005.

10. Asmae Fahmy, "For These 17 COVID Long Haulers, Reactivated Viruses May Be to Blame," Verywell Health, January 21, 2022.

11. "What Is ME?" #MEAction, accessed April 13, 2022, https://www.meaction.net/learn/what-is-me.

12. "Postural Orthostatic Tachycardia Syndrome," Dysautonomia International, accessed April 13, 2022, https://dysautonomiainternational.org/page.php?ID=30.

13. "Diagnosing MCAS," Mast Cell Action, accessed April 13, 2022, https://www.mastcellaction.org/diagnosing-mcas.

14. "What Are the Ehlers-Danlos Syndromes?," The Ehlers-Danlos Society, accessed April 13, 2022, https://www.ehlers-danlos.com/what-is-eds.

15. "Autoimmune Diseases," Cleveland Clinic, last modified July 21, 2021, https://my.clevelandclinic.org/health/diseases/21624-autoimmune-diseases.

16. Lauren Nichols, "Long Covid Diagnostic Tests," Long Covid Patient, last modified June 11, 2022, https://www.longcovidpatient.com/diagnostics.

CHAPTER 7: DOWN IN THE WELL, WE WILL MOURN AND SING

I. Maura Boldrini et al., "How COVID-19 Affects the Brain," *JAMA Psychiatry* 78, no. 6 (March 26, 2021): 682–83.

2. Gwenaelle Douad et al, "SARS-CoV-2 is associated with changes in brain structure in UK Biobank," *Nature* 604 (March 7, 2022): 697–707.

3. Boldrini et al., op. cit.

4. "Nearly One in Five American Adults Who Have Had COVID-19 Still Have 'Long COVID,'" Centers for Disease Control and Prevention, accessed July 18, 2022, https://www.cdc.gov/nchs/pressroom/nchs_press_releases/2022/20220622.htm.

5. "Long COVID," Centers for Disease Control and Prevention, accessed July 18, 2022, https://www.cdc.gov/nchs/covid19/pulse/long-covid.htm.

6. Leo Sher, "Post-COVID syndrome and suicide risk," *QJM: Monthly Journal of the Association of Physicians* 114, no. 2 (2021): 95–98.

7. "Small NIH study reveals how immune response triggered by COVID-19 may damage the brain," National Institute of Neurological Disorders and Stroke, July 5, 2022.

8. Joseph Altman et al., "Autoradiographic and histological evidence of postnatal hippocampal neurogenesis in rats," *Journal of Comparative Neurology* 124, no. 3 (June 1965): 319–35.

9. Eric Garland et al., "Neuroplasticity, Psychosocial Genomics, and the Biopsychosocial Paradigm in the 21st Century," *Health & Social Work* 34, no. 3 (August 2009): 191–99.

10. Monica Malowney et al., "Availability of Outpatient Care from Psychiatrists: A Simulated-Patient Study in Three U.S. Cities," *Psychiatric Services* 66, no. 1 (January 2015): 94–96.

II. Catherin K. Ettman et al., "Prevalence of Depression Symptoms in US Adults Before and During the COVID-19 Pandemic," *JAMA Network Open* 3, no. 9 (2020): e2019686.

12. Ibid.

13. "DSM-5 Diagnostic Criteria for PTSD," *Trauma-Informed Care in Behavioral Health Services* (Rockville, MD: Substance Abuse and Mental Health Services Administration, 2014).

14. Judith Lewis Herman, "Complex PTSD: A syndrome in survivors of prolonged and repeated trauma," *Journal of Traumatic Stress* 5, no. 3 (1992): 377–91.

15. "America's Mental Health 2018," Cohen Veterans Network, accessed April 13, 2022, https://www.cohenveteransnetwork.org/wp-content/uploads/2018/10/Research-Summary-10-10-2018.pdf.

CHAPTER 10: THE SEARCH FOR COMMUNITY

I. "Lockdown in India has impacted 40 million internal migrants: World Bank," *The Hindu*, April 23, 2020.

2. Padma Priya (@priyakamal), "5 days ago, i developed fever. it was low at first. 99 degrees. i had a bad headache that day. i popped a Dolo and kept working," Twitter, April 26, 2020, https://twitter.com/priyakamal/status/1254307706430607362?s=21&t=xU6GhHEYWAhXLQh75uhWiA.

3. Naranya Health, "Understanding Chikungunya Arthritis | Dr. Pradeep R Kumar," YouTube video, 3:59, February 28, 2020, https://www.youtube.com/watch?v=MiYqg63Po6c; Himanshu Pathak, Mithun C Mohan, and Vinod Ravindran, "Chikungunya Arthritis," *Clinical Medicine* 19, no. 5 (2019): 381–85.

CHAPTER II: KNOWLEDGE IS POWER

1. Lisa McCorkell et al., "Patient-Led Research Collaborative: embedding patients in the Long COVID narrative," *PAIN Reports* 6, no. 1 (2021): e913.

2. This list isn't exhaustive, but it covers some of the most important and common considerations. For more on how to review research studies, check out "Understanding Medical Research," MedlinePlus, last modified March 16, 2022, https://medlineplus.gov/understandingmedicalresearch.html; and Stephen D. Simon, "How to Read a Medical Journal Article," University of South Alabama Family Medicine Department, accessed April 14, 2022, http://www.fammed.usouthal.edu/Scholarly%20Activities/Activity1/HowToReadAJournalArticle—Abridged.pdf. There are also several free online courses that dive in deeper like the Patient-Centered Outcomes Research Institute's Research Fundamentals course.

3. Lindsey Konkel, "Racial and Ethnic Disparities in Research Studies: The Challenge of Creating More Diverse Cohorts," *Environmental Health Perspectives* 123, no. 12 (2015): A297.

4. Paula A. Johnson et al., "Sex-Specific Medical Research: Why Women's Health Can't Wait," Brigham and Women's Hospital, accessed April 14, 2022, https://www.brighamandwomens.org/assets/bwh/womens-health/pdfs/connorsreportfinal.pdf.

5. Nisreen A. Alwan, "Lessons from Long COVID: working with patients to design better research," *Nature Reviews Immunology* 22 (2022): 1–2.

6. Jessica T. Davis et al., "Cryptic transmission of SARS-CoV-2 and the first COVID-19 wave," *Nature* 600 (2021): 127–32.

7. "Estimated COVID-19 Burden," Centers for Disease Control, last modified November 16, 2021, https://www.cdc.gov/coronavirus/2019-ncov/cases-updates/burden.html.

8. Hannah E. Davis et al., "Characterizing long COVID in an international cohort: 7 months of symptoms and their impact," *eClinicalMedicine* 38 (2021).

9. Max Augustin et al., "Post-COVID syndrome in non-hospitalised patients with COVID-19: a longitudinal prospective cohort study," *Lancet Regional Health—Europe* 6 (2021).

10. Sabra L. Klein et al., "Sex, age, and hospitalization drive antibody responses in a COVID-19 convalescent plasma donor population," *Journal of Clinical Investigation* 130, no. 11 (2020): 6141–50.

11. Vasileios Nittas et al., "Long COVID Through a Public Health Lens: An Umbrella Review," *Public Health Review* 43, no. 1604501 (2022).

12. Hannah Davis et al., "Characterizing long COVID in an international cohort."

13. Ibid.

14. As of time of writing, Hannah Davis (@ahandvanish), PLRC (@patientled), Dr. Nisreen Alwan (@Dr2NisreenAlwan), and Dr. Eric Topol (@EricTopol) on Twitter; Lauren Nichols (@laurenthemedium) and LongCovidDoc (@longcoviddoc) on Instagram; and the Covid-19 Research Involvement Group on Facebook often break down the latest in Long COVID research. You can also look at existing research, especially on post-viral illness, on other organizations' websites. For example, #MEAction has a crowdsourcing encyclopedia called me-pedia.org that dives into a lot of research, and Dysautonomia International posts research summaries.

15. "Fair Market Calculator," National Health Council, accessed March 20, 2022, https://nationalhealthcouncil.org/fair-market-value-calculator.

16. A note about informal polls: When drafting the question-and-answer options, it's important to word them in an objective way that does not lead the respondent to a certain answer. Be careful about sharing these results publicly without giving the context and limitations of the poll.

17. Hannah Davis et al., "Characterizing long COVID in an international cohort."

18. Paul Wicks, "Patient, study thyself," *BMC Medicine* 16, no. 217 (2018).

CHAPTER 12: SUCH A POWERFUL LOVE

1. "All People with AIDS Are Innocent," Gran Fury, accessed April 13, 2022, https://www.granfury.org/all-people-with-aids-are-innocent.

AFTERWORD: THE FUTURE OF LONG COVID

1. Chen Chen et al., "Global Prevalence of Post-Coronavirus Disease 2019 (COVID-19) Condition or Long COVID: A Meta-Analysis and Systematic Review," *The Journal of Infectious Diseases* (2022): jiac136.

2. C.H. Sudre et al., "Attributes and predictors of long COVID," *Nature Medicine* 27 (2021): 626–31.

3. Hannah E. Davis et al., "Characterizing long COVID in an international cohort: 7 months of symptoms and their impact," *The Lancet* 38 (2021): 101019.

4. Ibid.

5. "The impact of COVID vaccination on symptoms of Long Covid: An international survey of 900 people with lived experience," https://www.longcovidsos.org/_files/ugd/8bd4fe_7301ed588cc44d1483e9fc8df7989a03.pdf?index=true.

6. Daisy Massey et al., "Change in Symptoms and Immune Response in People with Post-Acute Sequelae of SARS-Cov-2 Infection (PASC) After SARS-Cov-2 Vaccination," https://www.medrxiv.org/content/10.1101/2021.07.21.21260391v2.

7. "The Yale LISTEN Study," Yale School of Medicine, accessed June 20, 2022, https://medicine.yale.edu/ycci/listen-study.

8. Jan Choutka, et al., "Unexplained post-acute infection syndromes," *Nature Medicine* 28 (2022): 911–923.

Acknowledgments

This book was a truly collective effort: The project we've created would not have been possible without each and every contributor's perspective. But this book also could not have existed without the communities and people that supported and guided us through our illnesses, and our work writing about our experiences and raising awareness. We want to thank:

The team at Suno India; Rakesh Kamal; Pari; Eshwari & Nagarjuna; Krishna, Sumitra and Jayashree; The Robles family; Dr. Bojana Weatherly; Cognitive FX; Marguerite Wilder; William R Wilder; Bill Wilder; Gabriel, Sandra, and Guillermo Monterroso; Boris Gay; Jo Dainow; Letícia Soares; Fiona Lowenstein; Long COVID Support; Mimi Fox Melton; Team "Keep Karla Alive"; Faith R. Purnell; Sequoia Thompson; Dr. Lauren Ababio; Monica-Cole Fisher; Kimmy Campbell; Jerry Artukovich, Sherri Stephens, Robert Stephens, Anne McCloskey, Angela Laffin; professors and former classmates at the Goldman School of Public Policy; colleagues, staff, and students of NYU's department of Art & Public Policy; Alexandra Juhasz; Faith Idemundia; George Ayala; Tamara Oyola-Santiago; Lisa Hayeem Carver; Jaime Cortez; Thich Nhat Hanh; blood and chosen family who remain anonymous; Rose Perry; Erica Breyman; Laura Tabacof; Jamie Wood; Jenna Tosto-Mancuso; Sunik Kim; Sabrina Bleich; Angela Meriquez Vázquez; Christina Wright; Drew Lowenstein; Hannah Davis; Jennifer Brea; Ryan Prior; Lauren Nichols; Lily Silver, creator of How To Get On; disability lawyers Barbara Comerford and Cassie Springer Ayeni; Julie Reiskin, disability activist and executive director of Colorado Cross Disability Coalition; Ruth Castellanos, Long COVID activist in Canada; Dysautonomia International; Solve ME; Olivia Peluso, Margie Guerra, Besse Lynch, Jennifer Hergenroeder, Beth Bugler, Zach Pace, Joseph Payne, Aiden Blasi, and the team at The Experiment—your editorial guidance and overall support has been invaluable; The India Covid Survivors Group; The COVID-19 Longhauler Advocacy Project and Long COVID community; The Body Politic community; #MEAction staff and volunteers; the team at the Patient-Led Research Collaborative; the incredible leaders of Marked By Covid; the HIV community; radical and loving HIV movement groups including ACT UP Philadelphia, Positive Women's Network - USA, Health GAP, HIV

Racial Justice Now and the What Would an HIV Doula Do? collective; people with ME/CFS and other infection-initiated illnesses who have paved and guided the way for us; and all the authors of this book.

A few last words

"Thank you to the ones who stayed by my side, who kept me alive, hoping."
—Morgan Stephens

"Thank you to those who trusted me to share their stories."—Monique Jackson

"This project has broken my heart in a way that I sorely needed. This book will transcend what history will teach us about Long Covid in the decades to come."—Chimére L. Smith

"My chapter is about community, there are too many people to name, but you fought for my life then and now as I navigate disability—words will never be enough."—Karla Monterroso

"This project has given me the opportunity to speak my truth in a safe and supportive space. I never thought a chapter about my cognitive dysfunction could happen but it did with a great deal of love and care from the editors and my co-author! I'm forever grateful."—Terri Wilder

"'Never let a good crisis go to waste' has consistently been my guiding principle in my own recovery, and writing this book chapter has allowed me to disseminate information for others to build back their lives."—Rachel Robles

"I would like to thank Fiona for reaching out to me and asking me to write this chapter. It was therapeutic. I also want to thank Fiona and Olivia for the brilliant edits."—Padma Priya DVL

"I want to thank my son for being my rock and my drive."—Karyn Bishof

"As a person living with complex chronic conditions before Long COVID, I am so grateful to those newly joining our ranks who are vowing to fight for justice for all of us, and the disability justice movement for teaching us what we need to do to make it so."—JD Davids

"We dedicate our chapter in honor of Lily Silver, whose work creating the How To Get On website has helped so many people living with ME/CFS and associated conditions, including Long COVID, walk the difficult path of seeking financial support. We extend gratitude to the disabled activists who came before us, who have worked hard to change laws and make access easier for future generations of disabled people."—Alison Sbrana

"This work is true health advocacy in action—it has been a privilege to be included. Thank you."—David Putrino

"It is an honor to share with the world the culmination of knowledge and love that I've gained from the Patient-Led Research Collaborative, the Long COVID and associated conditions community, my former classmates and professors, and my friends and family."—Lisa McCorkell

"I am grateful to all of the early mentors who taught me to interrogate, investigate, and search beyond obvious headlines for hidden truths, and to everyone who encouraged me to trust my gut. I want to thank my grandparents and surrogate grandparents for teaching me to be nimble, fierce, creative, confident, cautious, and funny, even and especially during times of crisis; I know you'd be so proud (and so pissed) that this book exists. My work during this pandemic would not have been possible without the support of many fellow journalists and editors—especially freelancers and disabled and/or chronically ill journalists. To all the friends and family without Long COVID who educated themselves on it, I appreciate you. To every long-hauler who has ever trusted me with your story, thank you. To all my internet friends, you helped me forge a path in the wilderness; I'll never forget that."—Fiona Lowenstein

Resources

SUPPORT GROUPS

Body Politic | @itsbodypolitic

One of the very first COVID support groups, created by patients for patients in March 2020, is a moderated and channel-organized group on the private Slack chat platform. A global leader in Long COVID advocacy and research, Body Politic offers educational and social events, as well as research, media, and advocacy opportunities to all members. Open to anyone with prior COVID-19 infection and their caretakers.

Subgroups include: 70+ channels for body systems, demographics (BIPOC, LGBTQIA, Spanish speakers, medical professionals, teachers, etc.) and more
Technological difficulty: easy to moderate
Size: large (12K+ global members)

Black COVID-19 Survivors

A private Facebook group for Black COVID-19 survivors. From the group: "Black and African-American people have been hard hit by the COVID-19 pandemic during a time when we already face medical inequality and bias in diagnosis and treatment. Come share your story, your family's story and let's talk out what's needed for recovery and reducing the spread."
Technological difficulty: easy
Size: medium (1,700+ people)

#ME Action | @MEActNet

Offering a variety of private Facebook support groups for Long COVID and ME/CFS.
Subgroups include: support groups for Long COVID and ME/CFS, state chapters for location-specific support and activism, pregnancy and parenting with ME/CFS, caregiver support group, military and veteran families
Technological difficulty: easy
Size: small to medium

Dysautonomia International | @Dysautonomia

Offering a variety of private Facebook support groups for people with autonomic nervous system disorders. Dysautonomia can be common in people with Long COVID or ME/CFS.
Subgroups include: Facebook groups for all US states, as well as specific support groups for teens, college, LGBTQ+, Black community, and men
Technological difficulty: easy
Size: medium

COVID-19 Longhauler Advocacy Project | @C19LH_Advocacy

Offering a variety of private Facebook groups to create a space for advocacy, education, and support for people with Long COVID. A great space to get involved with activism. State chapters also offer small support groups to help you find resources in your area.
Subgroups include: Small Facebook groups for US states
Technological difficulty: easy
Size: medium (state chapters: small)

Long Covid Support - Facebook | @long_covid

A large private Facebook group offering support for Long COVID with international reach. This is a private group for people with Long COVID or people who are caring for someone with Long COVID.
Technological difficulty: moderate, due to size
Size: very large (50K+)

Long Covid Families | @LongCovidFam

Peer support and workshops for caregivers, children, and individuals with long-term complications from COVID-19. Spanish language support (particularly for teens and school accommodation support) in progress. Also offers guidance on accommodations at school and work.
Subgroups include: Spanish groups to come
Technological difficulty: easy
Size: small (100+ people)

Bateman Horne Center | @BatemanHorne

Twice monthly support Zooms facilitated by professionals. For individuals with ME/CFS, Long COVID, fibromyalgia, dysautonomia, and related chronic illnesses, as well as family members, friends, and care partners.
Technological difficulty: easy
Size: small

WEBSITES AND HOTLINES

U.S. Equal Employment Opportunity Commission: "What You Should Know about COVID-19 and the ADA, the Rehabilitation Act, and Other EEO Laws"
https://www.eeoc.gov/wysk/what-you-should-know-about-covid-19-and-ada-rehabilitation-act-and-other-eeo-laws

US Department of Health and Human Services Office for Civil Rights and US Department of Justice Civil Rights Division: "Disability Rights Section joint guidance on 'Long COVID' as a Disability Under the ADA, Section 504, and Section 1557"
https://www.ada.gov/long_covid_joint_guidance.pdf

No End in Sight Void: #NEISVoid is a hashtag started by Brianne Benness and used on Twitter for discussions on chronic illness, whether you have a diagnosis or not.
https://noendinsight.co/neisvoid-explained/

ACL Administration for Community Living: resources for COVID-19 related disabilities
ACL.gov

National Employment Lawyers Association: a registry of employment lawyers
https://exchange.nela.org/memberdirectory/findalawyer COVID-19

Longhauler Advocacy Project: "A Comprehensive Guide for COVID-19 Longhaulers and Providers"
https://docs.google.com/document/d/1FcmTJksCZS8TfinN_YVrqGeyShZIfer6RmbJTDu41k/edit COVID-19

Body Politic's resource page on Long COVID: includes tips for patients, caregivers, and clinicians
https://www.wearebodypolitic.com/resources

Job Accommodations Network (JAN)
https://askjan.org/

Substance Abuse and Mental Health Services Administration (SAMHSA) hotline: can get you answers to general mental health questions and help you locate services in your area.
1-800-662-HELP

Anxiety and Depression Association of America
adaa.org

Mental Health America
https://mhanational.org/

National Alliance on Mental Health
https://www.nami.org/Home

BLOGS/ARTICLES/PODCASTS/DOCUMENTARIES

Ed Yong's series on Long COVID in *The Atlantic*
"Covid-19 Can Last for Several Months," June 4, 2020
"Long-haulers Are Redefining COVID-19," August 19, 2020
"Long-haulers Are Fighting for Their Future," September 1, 2021
"Health-Care Workers with Long COVID Are Being Dismissed," November 24, 2021

How To Get On: a self advocacy guide, including easy-to-understand explanations of disability benefits, government assistance, and financial survival
https://howtogeton.wordpress.com/

***Unrest*: a documentary by #MEAction co-founder Jennifer Brea, which provides an excellent primer to ME/CFS. Especially recommended for caregivers, providers, and others looking to better understand.**

***Crip Camp*: a documentary chronicling the disability rights movement that advocated for historic legislation changes.**

Longhauler Advocacy Project: "Open Letter to President Biden and National Leadership"
https://www.longhauler-advocacy.org/open-letter

Sins Invalid: "10 Principles of Disability Justice"
https://www.sinsinvalid.org/blog/10-principles-of-disability-justice

***The Rest Room*: a podcast by Natasha Lipman that covers living well with chronic illness, through empathetic, informative and evidence-based guides on a whole host of topics like pacing, exercise, and chronic pain.**
http://natashalipman.com/podcast-home/

Index

external temperature regulation, 43
eyesight problems, 108

F

Facebook, support groups on, 41, 92, 204–5, 253
fainting/feeling faint, 18, 34, 37, 40, 133, 142, 203–5. *See also* vagus nerve
false negative testing, 77–81, 83
fatigue, recognizing, 22. *See also* symptoms
Federal Office for Civil Rights (US), 88
financial issues, 73–93
  anticipating, 74–76
  Centers for Independent Living and, 88, 89, 91–92
  compensation for patient representatives, 227
  diagnosing Long COVID and, 123–24
  difficulty of proving disability and, 76–85
  of disability justice, 242–44
  disabled community resources for, 86–87
  government assistance programs, 89–90
  health insurance and medical bills, 90
  research funding and, 220–21
  understanding disability rights for, 85–86, 87–88
  work accommodations and, 88–89
findings (research studies), 219–20
Florida, Department of Children and Families, 83
Fraser, Elizabeth, 168
Frey, Dennis, 69

G

gallbladder surgery, 52, 60–61, 63
gastrointestinal issues, 5, 6, 46
Gay, Boris, 185
Gay and Lesbian Health Conference (1983), 239

gender bias. *See* bias in health care
Google Scholar, 216
government assistance (US). *See also* resources and support
  Medicaid, 89–90
  Social Security Disability Insurance (SSDI), 83–84, 89–91, 180
Guidance on "Long COVID" as a Disability Under the ADA, Section 504, and Section 1557 (Federal Office for Civil Rights, US), 88
Guruprasad, Dr. (internist), 205
gut microbiome (dysbiosis), 140

H

"happy hypoxia," 20
headaches, 46
healing, defining, 9–10
health insurance
  diagnosis codes for, 123–24
  finding resources for, 90
  HIV and, 235
Health Resources and Services Administration (HRSA), 158
heart health issues
  coronary heart disease in women, 39
  dysautonomia and, 43–44
  tachycardia, 21, 23, 142, 204 (*see also* postural orthostatic tachycardia syndrome)
  testing for, 204
Hebert, Pato, 56
heparin-induced extracorporeal LDL precipitation (HELP-apheresis), 137
Herman, Judith, 156
herpes simplex virus 1 (HSV-1), 141
HIV/AIDS
  activism for, 172, 173, 226, 233–45 (*see also* disability justice)
  AIDS Coalition to Unleash Power (ACT UP), 7, 235
Hogan, Larry, 96

About the Contributors

KARYN BISHOF is the founder and president of the COVID-19 Longhauler Advocacy Project, a nonprofit whose mission is to advance the understanding of Long COVID and expedite solutions and assistance to long-haulers and their families through advocacy, education, research, and support. As a single mom, now disabled from a mild March 2020 infection while working as a firefighter paramedic, she advocates for millions through C-19LAP's work and serves on the NIH RECOVER Initiatives Ancillary Studies Oversight Committee and the Advisory Board of the Long COVID Research Fund.

JD DAVIDS, the founder of Strategies for High Impact (S4HI), is a queer and trans strategist, storyteller, and organizer living with multiple complex chronic conditions who is dedicated to national networks of disabled and chronically ill people, including people living with HIV, Long COVID, and ME/CFS. He also writes and hosts conversations for the *Cranky Queer Guide to Chronic Illness: Strategies for Health and Wellness for Sick Times.*

PATO HEBERT is an artist, teacher and organizer. He is a COVID long-hauler who tested positive in March 2020. His *Lingering* exhibition about long hauling debuted at Pitzer College in 2022. He serves as chair of the Department of Art & Public Policy at New York University's Tisch School of the Arts.

HEATHER HOGAN is the senior editor and social media director of Autostraddle, the largest website for LGBTQ women and non-binary people on the internet. She lives in New York City with her wife and their cackle of rescued pets. You can follow her work on Twitter @theheatherhogan.

MONIQUE JACKSON is a London-based artist and Long COVID advocate. She is the creator of The Still Ill Corona Diary, which documents her journey with experiencing Long COVID through an online graphic journal.

NAINA KHANNA (she/they) is the co-executive director of PWN-USA. A national speaker, trainer, and advocate, she has worked in the HIV field since 2005, following her HIV diagnosis in 2002. Prior to working in HIV, Naina cofounded and served as national field director for the League of Pissed Off Voters, a progressive national organization working to expand participation of young people and communities of color in electoral politics. She is currently pursuing a PhD in medical sociology at the University of California, San Francisco.

LISA MCCORKELL is a Long COVID patient advocate and cofounder of the Patient-Led Research Collaborative (PLRC). She has a background in writing, policy analysis, and advocacy, and has conducted quantitative and qualitative research on issues in public health, criminal justice, labor and employment, digital equity, and more. She has a master's in public policy from UC Berkeley and a bachelor of arts in political science from UCLA.

KARLA MONTERROSO is the founder and managing partner of Brava Leaders where she is a coach, strategist, and adviser for several organizations and people doing work impacted by the changing dynamics of the demographic shift. She supports their ability to distribute power strategically and contend with bridging the new divide between the social and institutional experiences of power. Karla has spent two decades focused on growing the people and program functions of rapidly scaling social enterprises driving youth advocacy and leadership.

DONA KIM MURPHEY is a neurologist, neuroscientist, historian of science, and community organizer. She organizes at the intersections of race, poverty, immigration, criminal (in)justice, and health. Understanding the interrelated health of individuals, our communities, and our democracy, Dona combats misinformation and disinformation as it pertains to COVID, has run for her local school board in Texas on a platform of whole child health, and cofounded Doctors in Politics. As a COVID long-hauler, she has learned to manage low energy and exercise much greater self-compassion in her pursuits.

PADMA PRIYA DVL is the cofounder and editor-in-chief at Suno India, an award-winning podcast platform. As an independent journalist, she has also written for leading media houses in India. She has also worked as an advocacy and communication specialist for the Nobel Peace Prize–winning organization

Doctors Without Borders. She has hosted multiple podcasts on underreported stories such as *Dear Pari*, on adoption; *The Suno India Show*, on current affairs; and *Pinjra Tod Kar*, on women empowerment, to name a few.

DAVID PUTRINO is a physical therapist with a PhD in neuroscience and is currently the director of rehabilitation innovation for the Mount Sinai Health System and an associate professor of rehabilitation and human performance at the Icahn School of Medicine at Mount Sinai. He has published over one hundred peer-reviewed scientific articles and book chapters and is the author of *Hacking Health: How to Make Money and Save Lives in the HealthTech World*, which is available from Amazon and Springer Nature. In 2019, he was named Global Australian of the Year for his contributions to health care.

YOCHAI RE'EM is a psychiatrist and psychotherapist practicing in New York City, where he contracted COVID in March of 2020, and where he has provided care to those with Long COVID–associated psychiatric issues. He has contributed to Long COVID research efforts as a patient-researcher member of Patient-Led Research Collaborative for COVID-19.

RACHEL ROBLES (she/her) is a Long COVID patient advocate based in Brooklyn, NY. After becoming ill in March 2020, she joined Body Politic and the Patient Led Research Collaborative (PLRC), where she helps disseminate information from leading researchers to patients. Rachel is currently a senior data strategist and holds a bachelor's degree in operations research engineering from Cornell University.

ALISON SBRANA (she/her) is a disability activist based in Fort Collins, Colorado, living with complex chronic illness caused by a viral infection in 2014. She is passionate about helping chronically ill people navigate disability rights, medical care, and benefits as a former care coordinator for Colorado's Medicaid program. Alison is actively involved with direct peer support and policy advocacy as a board member of Body Politic, a health justice organization working to break down barriers to patient-driven, whole-person care through a global network of COVID-19 patients, chronic illness allies, and disability advocates.

CHIMÉRE L. SMITH is an award-winning middle school teacher in Baltimore who, since June 2020, has acted as a writer, thought leader, and media and guest panelist on international and national platforms, using her voice and personal experiences to bring awareness to the economic, psychological, and physical devastation of Long COVID on urban communities. As one of the first Black women with Long COVID, Smith has shared her story with PBS, MSNBC, CBS, CNN, *The New York Times*, and *The Washington Post*. Coined as "passionate" by state and local government officials, she was personally chosen to testify before Congress, offering greater awareness of the often-overlooked plight of Black, disabled, and low-income women in America. Today, Smith serves as a guest speaker, moderator, and writer for health and social organizations who seek a unique, independent, and diverse presence to educate and encourage other minority Long COVID sufferers. She is a board member of Body Politic and a featured writer in HuffPost.

LETÍCIA SOARES is a biologist, scientist, and educator. She earned a master's in ecology from the Instituto Nacional de Pesquisas da Amazônia (Brazil) and a PhD in biology from the University of Missouri-St. Louis (USA). She was a postdoctoral scholar when she became disabled by COVID-19 while living in Ontario, Canada. Currently, she lives on the land of the Pataxo Indigenous people, in the state of Bahia in northeast Brazil.

MORGAN STEPHENS is a freelance journalist and production assistant with CNN. Her writing and reporting has appeared in CNN Opinion, CNN Politics, HuffPost, and *The Washington Post*. She's writing a book on Long COVID, in which she'll detail her experience and report on how the US addresses the public health crisis.

TERRI L. WILDER, MSW, is an award-winning social worker, writer, and activist focused on disability justice for people living with HIV, Long COVID, and myalgic encephalomyelitis (ME). She was diagnosed with ME in March 2016. Since her diagnosis, she has worked with elected officials, public health departments, health care providers, and activists across the globe. She is currently a consultant for #MEAction and has represented the organization on the federal Chronic Fatigue Syndrome Advisory Committee (CFSAC). Terri is also a journalist with TheBodyPro (thebodypro.com), a website supporting the HIV/AIDS workforce.

About the Editor

FIONA LOWENSTEIN (they/them) is an award-winning independent journalist, producer, and speaker covering health justice, wellness culture, gender, sexuality, and the media. Their writing has been published in *The New York Times*, *Teen Vogue*, *Vox*, *The Guardian*, *Business Insider*, and the *Columbia Journalism Review*, among other publications. In 2018, Fiona founded the queer feminist wellness collective and events series Body Politic, which is now a grassroots patient-led health justice organization. In the spring of 2020, Fiona wrote what seems to be the first mainstream media account of what we now call Long COVID in *The New York Times* and cofounded the Body Politic Covid-19 Support Group. Fiona speaks regularly on news programs, podcasts, and at events and has served as a subject matter expert on Long COVID for the NIH, CDC, WHO, and POTUS Covid-19 Health Equity Task Force, among other health agencies. They have been covering COVID-19 patient issues as a journalist and writer for the past two years and have produced a series of work meant to help other journalists navigate reporting on these topics. Fiona currently lives in Los Angeles with their partner.

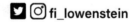 fi_lowenstein

CPSIA information can be obtained
at www.ICGtesting.com
Printed in the USA
LVHW051359170623
750034LV00007B/10